SLEEP TRAINING THE BREASTFED BABY (OR NOT)

Sophia Felder FNP IBCLC

CONTENTS

INTRODUCTION

This book aims to integrate knowledge about lactation, infant sleep patterns, mental health, and hunger hormones. The knowledge shared here will help parents who are feeding infants and toddlers be empowered to make decisions that are safe and will work for their family. Each family is respected as an autonomous unit that needs to make decisions that work for their lifestyle, culture, and preferences.

I firmly believe that knowledge is empowering. The more you know about a topic the more likely you are to succeed at doing it, and feel good about the outcome and the journey. The steep learning curve that happens when you have your first baby is currently too steep, especially for sleep deprived and vulnerable new parents. My aim in writing this book (and my other books) is to flatten that learning curve and bring more education to the general public.

Nursing and getting sleep are often at odds with one another, but they do not have to be. Using data we have on biological optimization for sleeping and eating, we can bio-hack routines to be more sustainable. This will make room for a longer and more enjoyable lactation relationship for many parents.

Many sleep training methods are at odds with a parent's intuition, and can sabotage milk supply and nursing relationships. Some sleep training methods have also been shown through studies to be unhealthy long term for baby's emotional and mental health, particularly ones that leave babies alone to cry un-soothed for extended periods of time. Many parents sleep train and then wonder why nursing is no longer going well, because the sleep training does not take into consideration the needs of lactation. Rather than having dyads come to me to fix what the sleep consultant broke, I would prefer to educate parents on how to protect their lactation, consider infant needs and norms, while simultaneously getting more rest. I would not say any of my suggestions are "sleep-training" in the traditional sense of the phrase. The knowledge I present will, however, help you go into choosing to sleep-train (or not) from a more informed space.

This book serves to promote lactation relationship longevity through avoiding premature weaning based on lack of sleep. If a parent wants to breastfeed longer but feels helpless due to lack of knowledge on how to get more sleep, they face a tumultuous dilemma. My aim is to make the relationship less burdensome while introducing minimal interference to the long-term goals of the dyad, and with consideration of minimizing safety risks. I focus on night-time sleep, not especially napping. This book is not all encompassing of everything there is to know about infant sleep, but is mostly about its relationship to lactation.

Our nursing initiation rates are high, but continuation rates are low--and I am sure that part of this trend is lack of sleep for parents, but it doesn't have to be. I believe through education we can change that, and I hope this is what my books do. Many of the topics covered in this book are expanded upon, in addition to many other concerns, in my general lactation education book titled "Can I talk you out of breastfeeding?" This is another awesome resource for parents, and is a cheeky way to ask you a deep question. If I lay out the truth, will you still try? Trust me, it's worth a read, and is a great gift for expectant parents (and the reviews reflect this)!

About Me:

On a personal level, I have endured many challenges with breastfeeding, including enduring months of sleep deprivation. I believe that my breastfeeding problems were a gift to me. I have a heart of service and want to use my gifts to help others. I deeply and personally know how it is such a vulnerable and special time, and how the decisions around infant feeding and sleep can feel so heavy.

Professionally, I am a Family Nurse Practitioner and an Internationally Board-Certified Lactation Consultant. I have a Bachelor of Science in Psychology, Bachelor of Science in Nursing, and Master of Science in Nursing. I have worked in Maternal-Infant Health since 2012, and lactation support has always been part of my work; in 2018 I decided to make lactation medicine a focus of my practice.

I work full time as a Family Nurse Practitioner, and have specialty knowledge in lactation. I see patients on the Olympic Peninsula in Washington State, and do online consulting. In between work and parenting I educate and connect with my readers and patients through my Instagram and Facebook, both found via @thelactationpractitioner. This is also where you can find information on how to book with me and purchase my other books.

For the greater part of the last decade of my life countless parents have expressed gratitude and appreciation for my candor and for educating them, so I figured I have something to offer on a larger scale. I have written, and am writing, other books to help educate parents about many of the challenges of lactation and modern parenting. My general lactation education book "Can I talk you out of breastfeeding?" is a tongue-in-cheek title (so, not actually trying to talk you out of it) that has the educational material modern parents are actually craving. I was moved to write because I was repeatedly upset at hearing parents felt unprepared for the realities of lactation (or infant feeding in general) and I seek to change the conversations we have around lactation and the mental health of new parents through my writing. I cover topics no other lactation book dares. Much like this book covers many considerations that lactation or sleep training books leave out. I look at biological norms, biological data feedback, all the options, and then I look at the lactating parent and the infant as a whole and then again as separate units. My books are more than how to manuals, and give real and practical information. Mental health is at the forefront of my books and my aim is to empower parents to make the best personalized decisions for their families from an informed space. Resources for when you hit snags are also included in each book.

In clinical practice and in my writing, I strive to provide evidence-based care, and sometimes all that I have is anecdotes. This is the current reality of the fast-paced world we live in. I do my best to balance it all, and use my best clinical judgement.

Given all that information, I believe that I can help new parents. I want to help, and to help parents through this time is my honor.

Disclaimer:

This book is intended for educational and entertainment purposes only and does not replace medical advice following a thorough and detailed assessment by an appropriately credentialed provider. Reading this book does not establish a patient-provider relationship. The author disclaims any liability of outcomes based on the information provided in this book and expects all readers needing professional assistance to seek it in a timely and appropriate manner.

WHY IT MATTERS

It can be challenging to deal with an abrupt change in lifestyle for a new and lactating parent. Additionally, these changes can affect a relationship with a partner. Cluster feeding, leaking, lack of sleep, growth spurts, teething, engorgement, and being the primary caretaker are just some of those challenges, and the challenges begin right away.

To sleep train or not is not as black and white as many make it out to be, and there are many different versions of sleep training. In reality, it is something parents do to get more sleep so it needs a nuanced in-depth exploration, especially as it pertains to lactation.

Many parents believe they have to sleep train, and that it is a rite of passage or a necessary part of parenting. Not only is this not true, but it can also sabotage nursing relationships that were otherwise going well, and cause a lot of needless stress for parents who were otherwise doing fine without sleep training. Knowing there are other options or more gentle approaches to facilitating more rest is part of a complete education on these topics, and education is empowering.

In a typical parent-child relationship, the parent who is lactating has a severe sleep deficit when they are waking frequently for night feedings. A completely normal part of taking care of a newborn is how the lack of sleep can affect a person. Parents do not get much sleep when they have a newborn, less if nursing does not go well. Babies are just very disruptive to sleep. In general when we are exhausted, our physical and mental health is negatively impacted. Being exhausted just does not feel good.

Our exhaustion can make us edgy and negative. You may resent your baby when they wake more than usual at night. You also might resent your partner for sleeping through midnight feeds. Often when we are tired, we are snappier and more emotionally labile. During postpartum, the body and the soul are under a lot of pressure, meeting seemingly constant demands. Learning to adjust and grow with these big changes is really challenging, and its typical to have a hard time during this period.

What I just went over, obviously, can influence your relationships with others. Especially the people who live with us. Sleep deprivation can make that extra few minutes to spare seem like it should only be made available for a nap, and you would prioritize this over spending it being intimate with a partner or taking time to call a friend. The sheer exhaustion and workload of parenthood can make it hard to have time to get in the mood, and exacerbate feelings of overstimulation, and being "touched-out." When we get a moment alone, we might crave to avoid stimulation of any kind. We lose time and energy to connect with our loved ones in the ways we used to.

Of utmost importance is the effect sleep deprivation has on our mental health. Parents often expect to hold onto their joy and elation every moment of the postpartum experience. This can feel very jarring and incongruent with the reality of being exhausted and overwhelmed by their newborn. Then there is the self-shame for feeling this, which can lead to deeper and more consistent negative emotions. It is okay to not enjoy every moment or have moments of doubt and even negative feelings about having become a parent. At the same time, we may go in and out of feeling high on the love we have for our infant. When we are sleep deprived and struggling, this push and pull is normal. This risk can be true of all parents, of course, but especially optimistic, and high-achieving personalities.

Extreme sleep deprivation is also a risk factor and exacerbation factor for mood disorders. Common thoughts of parents who are struggling with mood imbalances are "Something has got to give," or "I don't feel like myself," or "I feel stuck," or "I am failing at this." You might experience suicidal thoughts, not feel connected to your baby, be overwhelmed easily, or feel you are a burden to your family. You might have trouble trusting your instincts or recognizing them. Many people experience physical discomfort as well as sadness, an urge to cry, loss of enjoyment of foods and hobbies, difficulty sleeping or wanting to sleep more than usual, feeling unmotivated, and lacking the energy or motivation to maintain usual hygiene habits. These can be clues that you might have Postpartum Depression (PPD) or Postpartum Anxiety (PPA), and it is time to seek help.

Sometimes our PPD or PPA symptoms manifests as rage, or you might be experiencing a mood disorder only recently starting to be recognized called Postpartum Rage (PPR). You might find yourself losing control and yelling, even over minor things. You might struggle to tap into your patience, empathy, and logic. This is usually followed by a deep sense of regret and guilt, and leaves you wondering why you are lacking self-control with your anger. Often this can be a sign that you are taking on too much, and not honoring the postpartum rest and recovery that your body is needing. Although, this is not always the case. These signs can mean it is time to seek help with your PPD/PPA/PPR with more logistical support, a healthcare assessment, counseling, or medications. It is important to note these postpartum conditions can happen even when a parent is well rested and supported, as well.

The highest risk factor for an episode of postpartum psychosis is an extended period of lack of sleep, and it can lend to the development of all of the other mood disorders. It starts with exhaustion, which leads to delusions, and then there are hallucinations, which walks us into the psychosis. Prioritizing sleep is so important, and often not given enough attention or consideration when planning for the time frame when new parents are in the throes of newborn life. If you do not set yourself up to get some sleep, you will actually have a harder time falling asleep the more over-tired you are. If you do not sleep enough for several days in a row, you can have a psychotic episode and need hospitalized. This can happen independently of being in a postpartum state. A postpartum psychosis can also happen without sleep deprivation. This scenario where sleep deprivation plays a role can sometimes be prevented with help from your healthcare team and support circle. Work with your healthcare team and the people who are living with you to make a safe-sleep plan. If you find that you are unable to sleep, you need to tell your healthcare provider.

There is help available for all mood disorders. You can seek support groups, go to counseling, take herbs, take medications, or any combination of these options. Your healthcare provider can do bloodwork to see if you have any fatiguing conditions like hypothyroidism or anemia, and then treat them. Your team can help you find supportive resources for logistical things that are stressors, and help you work out what can be let go of temporarily to ease your burdens. They might also help you find the words and the courage to ask your loved ones for more help. There are many safe medications, herbs, and treatments that can work well with lactation. Plus, you have the option of utilizing a lactation consultant to address your lactation challenges and worries head-on. Of course, I do hope this book also helps you get some more rest so you can improve that aspect of your health, which typically helps improve mental health.

If you are prone to mental illness or it runs in your family then it is a good idea to set up safety nets and support systems before you reach your postpartum period. Even parents with all the support in the world and all the sleep they crave can still develop postpartum mood disorders, because it is largely hormonally driven. It is always wise to be realistic and prepare for the possibilities, regardless of risk factors. Please do not anticipate that sleep training will cure a mood disorder. For some parents sleep training exacerbates mood disorders, especially methods that involve hearing your infant crying for long periods. I go much more in depth on lactation and mood disorders in my lactation book, if you want more information this is a great resource.

In addition to our mental health and relationships with others, this information is critical in helping parents reach their lactation goals and in feeling confident in their parenting decisions. Goals and expectations are usually in line with healthcare suggestions and guidelines, but parents lack the support and education needed to reach those goals. It shouldn't be a surprise to new parents what biological norms are for their own bodies or their infant's bodies. While getting completely adequate rest might be unachievable with an infant, we can aim to improve things so that the journey to reach those goals are at least sustainable, and not causing risks to our well-being or relationships with others.

This topic also matters because of the potential effects on the infant. Many sleep training methods interfere with the typical nursing dyad relationship, undermining the biological needs of the child. Some studies have shown negative effects of some sleep training methods on emotional and mental health, and adding a layer of dramatically interrupting the needs that are met through the nursing relationship is likely not going to have only positive impacts for the infant. This is especially true of methods that require separation or leaving the infant when they are upset. Of note, however, I must address the myth that sleep interruptions are bad for your infant or causing them to suffer—on the contrary this is the biological norm and infants sleep needs are very different from adult sleep needs.

There is also risk to the biological norms of the lactation process when we disrupt the feeding and sleeping cues of an infant. I discuss supply building and regulation in detail, and in relationship to sleep patterns, in order to explain the science behind why some sleep training methods can potentially cause clogs and mastitis for some parents, as well as a lowered milk supply and thus poor weight gain in an infant. I also explain how for some lactating parents, there are ways around this, or at least how to minimize impacts.

I believe the method I have come up with minimizes and mitigates all of these risks. By combining a method that is responsive to the infant but takes advantage of our knowledge of the body we can get parents more rest without compromising the nursing goals, the infant's needs, nor risk causing harm to their emotional or mental health. If after reading through you still decide doing anything to adjust your infant's sleep isn't for you, that is okay too! My goal for this book isn't to promote or diss sleep training, just educate. I do cover lots of other ways to facilitate rest, in addition to or instead of trying to change your infant's habits.

LACTATION AND SLEEP, PATTERNS AND NORMS

Many people interested in this book will be beyond pregnancy and the newborn phase, but I am including it for background knowledge, and for future considerations if you have more babies. I do cover some of the newborn norms of sleep, so it is helpful background information. Feel free to skim or skip this if you want to get to the more pressing information to your current situation. Much of this section is organized by age, so you can choose to focus in on what age range your baby is.

The beginning of lactation starts in pregnancy, so I start there. You start making colostrum while you are still pregnant, and you might leak! Colostrum is the precursor to mature milk (but is still milk) and has many immunity and nutritional benefits. Your milk transitions from colostrum to mature milk a few days after the baby is born, and the process is triggered by the delivery of the placenta. This is followed by some dramatic and sudden hormone changes. This transition from colostrum to mature milk is usually made apparent because of the engorgement phase, and for a few days the milk is "transitional." When you hear the phrase "my milk came in" this is the period to which most people are referring.

Between the infant's arrival earth-side and the milk "coming in" your baby will go through a few phases of sleeping and eating. Babies usually nurse 1 or 2 times after delivery before sleeping for a long stretch, because being born is hard work! Once they rest, they go on to eat every few hours for maybe a day or so, and then they go on a feeding frenzy. The baby has many messages that it needs to signal to your body through that seemingly non-stop feeding session, as well as some crying. The body needs to be made aware that the baby has now been born and has left the uterus; they survived the delivery, and they are vigorous enough that the body should start making milk for them in anticipation of their continued survival. While this sounds a little harsh, it is basic anatomy and physiology for mammals.

Many parents and postpartum healthcare workers call this signaling "second night syndrome." The baby seems ravenous on the second night, and the feeding parent gets very little sleep. Do not let this scare you, it is not like this long term, and it does not mean your baby is starving.

The baby, while in utero, swallows amniotic fluid. The amniotic fluid in their belly and the colostrum they drink are enough to keep them hydrated and keep their blood sugar stable until more milk is flowing, in most cases. They also have mostly brown fat, adults have mostly yellow. Brown fat burns more readily and so the baby uses those brown fat stores for energy while waiting for the milk to come in. Thus, a little bit of weight loss is an expectation during this time.

You will likely be encouraged to wake the baby at least every few hours, and they might be sleepy or alternatively feeding more frequently than expected. The thing is, newborns are baby animals and they can't tell time. They will signal when they need to go to the breast, and it will be in a seemingly erratic pattern. We rarely go wrong when we follow their lead. Their motto the first few weeks is: "If I am awake, I am eating." The reason we encourage them to eat at least every few hours is to help keep them hydrated and to help keep their blood sugar stable. This is a minimum of how often they should eat, not a maximum. This also helps protect and boost your supply. Your sleep, and theirs, will be broken and random. If ever there was a time to "sleep when the baby sleeps" it is the first few days of their life. I would even recommend doing this the first few weeks.

Some infants are at risk of being too sleepy to eat often enough, so we cannot follow their lead. If you are unsure if you should be waking your baby to eat, just error on the side of caution and do it until you get the all-clear from someone who knows if the baby is ready to take the lead or not (like an IBCLC). Complications, exceptions, and nuances in this process are explored in more detail in my lactation book.

Barring complications or exceptions, after the milk transitions babies sometimes go on a second feeding frenzy because their suckling is rewarded with more volume. Knowing what the process typically looks like can help avoid stressors and missteps, so I will expand on that. Babies will eat an average of 8 to 12 times in 24 hours. It will not be a nice neat every 2-hour schedule. They often want to nurse every 5 to 60 minutes when cluster feeding, or every 2 to 3 hours for the longer stretches between feeds. The total in the 24 hours will be somewhere between 8 to 12 for most days. With some variation you might expect that some babies some days eat only 6 times, and some babies some days eat 15 times. Whether the frequency or pattern is abnormal enough to warrant intervention will be determined by hydration status (monitored by counting wet and poopy diapers per day) and growth patterns (monitored by checking the baby's weight every few days or every couple of weeks). When in doubt, seek a professional out! Frequency can be influenced by infant preference, as well as mammae capacity and refill rate (more on that later). Gradually as the milk supply is more established your baby will stop cluster feeding so often and go for longer stretches between feeds more consistently.

Sleep-wake cycles often mirror milk volume ebb and flow in the early postpartum weeks. Prolactin is higher at night, so there is more milk volume, and babies will eat more at night. Babies are also still more comfortable with a dark quiet environment, like the womb. They do eventually adjust to be awake more during the day. You can gently encourage this transition by having the environment at a normal light and noise level all day, and keeping everything dark and quiet at night. Minimize playing and stimulation at night, and save it for the daytime.

Not removing the milk often enough or efficiently enough in the early postpartum days can be detrimental to supply, and letting a baby sleep several long stretches per day can be dangerous to their health. It is best to drain the breast as much as possible at least every 2-3 hours and to have no more than a single occurrence of a longer stretch than that every 24 hours. Generally, we can get away with one stretch of 4 to 6 hours for rest. The baby will still need to eat while we rest, until they are old enough and gaining weight well enough that their stabilization is no longer a concern. For most full-term infants that is when they have returned to their birth weight, and are about 2 weeks old. Once they are cleared to do so, they can also have a 3 to 6 hour stretch of rest without being woken to feed. Until then, you can pump or hand express once per day to have milk ready for a family member or caregiver to give the baby while you rest a longer stretch.

The mammae feeling full after engorgement resolves is actually a sign that they are not being drained well, or often enough. If we have repeated occurrences of full breasts the body gets the signal that we do not want or need that much milk, and it starts to make less. So, while it can be tempting to let the baby (and thus you) sleep several longer stretches per day, this can be detrimental to building your milk supply. If you are hybrid feeding with donor milk or formula and don't mind not having a full supply or already know you want or need to supplement, then it's okay to adjust your relationship based on that.

There can be a point where you supplement too often or too much, and it sacrifices so much of your supply that it dries up. So, if you are going to combo feed, be sure it involves a professional to help balance the milk sources and still protect your overall supply.

The mammae should soften after the engorgement period, and feel softer still, after each feeding; feeling fuller only briefly right before the next feeding as they have refilled between feeds. After supply regulation around 12 weeks the breasts continue to get flatter and have an even less full feeling. This is because the mammae transition from being a storage warehouse, where milk is always ready to feed with some extra to spare, to more of a feed on demand factory where the milk is made and pulled out of the breast as the infant nurses and requests it. The mammae are never empty because the milk making is on a slow and continual process, so even if a baby nurses for a long time and the breast feels soft there is still milk coming, it is just at a slower rate than at the beginning of the feed. These changes are normal and expected, and you can check in with your lactation consultant if the changes worry you. Education on low supply and how to define it and trouble shoot it can be found in my lactation book.

As both breasts start to fill with mature milk, when you offer the first breast and it is its most full, then the initial 2-3 let-downs every 2-3 minutes are a fast flow and the baby gets most of the volume in the first 5-6 minutes. They will keep nursing past that to get more milk and to seek comfort. While on the first breast the baby dozes off as the rate of flow slows down. This does not mean they are done, or full. The baby will have gotten to the fatty hindmilk and drained the breast well if they are starting to doze off. This is when you should at least offer the second side. When parents mistake the first dozing signs as being done or full they often find themselves frustrated or surprised when the baby wakes up 5 to 10 minutes later rooting for the breast. When you rouse them after getting sleepy on the first breast and then offer the second breast, they get the faster flowing milk again, and are happy to drink more. This is how a baby can potentially get more volume spending 10-15 minutes on each breast, rather than 20-30 minutes on one breast. This is also how you can possibly avoid having so many nursing sessions clustered together (though not entirely avoid cluster feeding). Doing this is not only beneficial to supply regulation but also reduces engorgement discomfort as well as baby's risks of jaundice, weight loss, inadequate gain, and poor blood sugar stabilization. They will still have cluster feeding sessions, no doubt, but less of them. This often translates to more sleep.

Once supply is more established and capacity determined,

you might find that your baby needs only one breast because each of your mammae has the capacity to hold the volume of a full feed. You would in that case want them to finish the feed on one side to ensure they got to the fatty hind milk. This can be confusing or hard to guess if your baby needs one or both sides, so do not be afraid to go check in with a consultant to clarify what would be best for you and your baby. There is no good blanket advice that will work for everyone, such as "10-15 minutes on each breast," because there is so much variation in capacity of breasts and efficiency of infants. Worrying about foremilk hindmilk balance and how it relates to offering both breasts usually only comes up if babies are struggling to gain weight, having severe gastrointestinal symptoms, or if a parent has an over-supply; so it is not something that most parents will have to worry about.

I am going to go more in depth here on comparing breastmilk amounts to formula amounts, because it often sabotages many lactation relationships when parents think they should be producing as much breastmilk as a formula fed baby eats. It also undermines many nursing relationships when nursing infants' sleep and eating patterns are compared to formula fed infants' sleep and eating patterns.

Formula fed babies usually eat larger quantities but less often, due to it digesting more slowly in the stomach and the tendency of bottle-fed infants to take larger quantities versus nursed infants. The amount they need continues to increase because formula is not a living substance that changes, like breastmilk. When babies get breast milk their intake is more constant, and as their gut matures, they become more efficient at absorbing more of the nutritional content. As the months go by, the proteins and other nutrition in the breastmilk also change to better suit the baby's needs. Additionally, babies who bottle feed tend to take larger volumes than those fed at breast, because at the breast they have more control and variation in the flow rate (this is true even when babies switch from months of exclusively pumped breastmilk back to the breast directly). Over time formula amounts tend to increase more than breastmilk volume. A formula fed baby might be taking 8 ounces per feed between 6-12 months, but a breast-milk fed baby should never do this. Occasionally, I see babies that want maybe 6 ounces per feed of breastmilk and do well with that, but most will stay in the 2.5 to 5-ounce range. The formula fed baby eats less often and sleeps longer stretches because the digestion of another species' milk proteins over-rides or delays some of their human biological drives to seek breastmilk more frequently. These are drives that serve to protect milk supply, and protect them from SIDs (Sudden Infant Death Syndrome), so it is not exactly a good thing to aim to over-ride it in the quest for more sleep. Formula feeding does not increase the risk of SIDs, and many people find that confusing but breastmilk being protective does not make the formula make SIDs more likely. There are great thorough explanations for this online if you want more detail. The amount of sleep gained is not usually statistically significant, and babies who get all formula tend to still wake 8-12 times per day to feed in the first few months, and go through cluster feeding during growth spurts, just like breastfed babies.

The first 2-4 months are little erratic, and by design. Getting on a schedule or focusing on sleep training can be detrimental to long term lactation success if not handled right. The reduction of baby's cluster feeding patterns coincides with our milk regulation hormonal patterns, first around 6 weeks and then again around 12 weeks. The erratic nursing pattern, or lack of a real pattern, is how the baby works with your body in tandem to continue to boost the supply the first 6-12 weeks. The cluster feeding and the sporadic nursing keep the breasts at a low volume compared to capacity, and this is what signals to the body to keep increasing the supply. Conversely, a full breast sends hormonal signals to lower supply. A full breast signals "Hey body, I don't need this much milk." This is why most lactation professionals discourage parents from putting a breastfed baby on a schedule. This is lo-gistically challenging, as it makes planning around nursing tricky when there is lack of a schedule. As their schedule regulates or be-comes more predictable so does the milk, because your body starts to get the signal that the baby is more content. After around 12 weeks it would be less risky to the lactation relationship to try to encourage a schedule.

If they never seem satisfied the first 4 to 6 weeks, it is because it is their job to act that way. This is part of the design of boosting the supply. Even bottle-fed babies will try to follow these instincts and cluster feed frequently the first 4-6 weeks. Obviously, with frequent feeding comes frequent waking. Their behavior, as such, is not the best or only indicator of adequate milk supply or transfer. The best indicators are diaper output and weight gain, and you can combine this data with signs of satiety after feeds to know if your baby is getting enough volume to thrive.

Even if it seems they are never satisfied, it is important to note that at times they actually are. To know if a baby is sometimes content, you will see their body give you clues. If they are truly never content, this might be a red flag and cause for concern. A content baby usually has open and relaxed hands, gets sleepy and drowsy at the breast after 10-15 minutes or more of nursing, their sucking starts to slow down, and they have good diaper output and weight gain. If they are nursing 30-45 minutes and coming off crying and upset, they may not be getting enough. This would also mean that you and the baby are not getting enough restful sleep.

Knowing normal diaper output, as well as weight, growth and sleep patterns will help you determine if your baby is getting enough nutrition and hydration. To be safe it would be wise to have a third party, preferably a non-biased professional, assess this for you. Even when we have data in front of us, our bias can cause us to deny that there is a problem present. Conversely, you knowing what is normal can help you advocate for yourself and your child with a professional, if you know something is off.

Ranges of normal for feeding frequency can be a big clue to whether or not baby is getting enough to eat, so be sure to note down somewhere how long and how often your baby is nursing. Frequent feeding does not mean they are not satisfied, and they will cluster feed even when their stomach is very full. This is ingrained and instinctive behavior that encourages the milk supply to keep increasing, and sometimes precedes a longer stretch of sleep. Cluster feeding tends to happen in the early evening when supply naturally dips and babies are over-tired and over-stimulated from a long day. The milk is fattier when there is lower volume and might help the baby sleep a longer stretch after the evening cluster session. Cluster feeding may also happen between midnight and five in the morning due to the abundance of milk flow and baby's instincts to night-feed. This helps them get large volumes of milk and it serves to stimulate the daily prolactin amounts, and thus overall daily milk production.

The first 2-3 months is also the Period of Purple Crying, which is when babies cry for extended periods, usually in the evening, it seems unrelated to anything or unexpected, they might appear they are in pain, it peaks around 6-8 weeks, and resolves around 12 weeks. There is excellent information online about PURPLE crying, and if you are unfamiliar, I encourage you to look it up. This can also be called "the witching hour," although it typically can last several hours. This time is also often very disruptive to rest.

As the baby gets older, they will change their patterns. This is especially true when they are ready to drop a nap every few months, and the feeding pattern will adjust. This is a time many parents worry about the supply changing, and there is no need. The body will adjust to the baby's new schedule. You do not ever need to force a change to nap schedules, babies and toddlers will nap as often as they need to meet their personal sleep requirements. You can, however, encourage naps when your child seems ready to rest. Paying attention to the time frame your baby is typically happy to be awake and then when they are ready to nap, and then helping facilitate that, helps prevent problems from over-tiredness like being fussy or resisting a nap. Babies that get enough naps during the day are usually better sleepers at night, and each child's needs are unique so it is something you have to watch and learn about them. Watching them closely you can learn what their early signs are of becoming tired.

How frequently your older infant nurses will partially depend on your capacity. Since most babies eat anywhere from 19-30 ounces per day, it also depends on their individual needs. Mammae that can hold 2-3 ounces at a time will often correspond with a baby that continues to nurse 8 times in 24 hours. That can come out to around up to 24 ounces per 24 hours. Mammae that have a larger capacity might correspond with a baby nursing only 6 times in 24 hours, because they are drinking a larger quantity less often. For example, if capacity is 5-6 ounces at a time and the baby eats 6 times that could be roughly 30 ounces per 24 hours. This will also depend on how well they take to solids around 6 months. Infant changes to nursing and milk intake in response to adding solids is very varied, and it does not tend to change sleep patterns. For example, more solids does not equate to more sleep. After around 12 months supply is much more stable and less sensitive to sleep pattern adjustments. The supply is then more regulated by supply and demand in-the-moment, and longer stretches without nursing are better tolerated. The first 12 months supply is very hormonally mediated and dependent on night time removal as well as frequent removal. I do go a lot more in depth on these lactation norms in my lactation book if you are someone who likes more detail.

TYPICAL SLEEP PATTERNS OF INFANTS AND TODDLERS

Let us be honest, you do not get much sleep with a newborn regardless of feeding methods. In fact, it is typical for sleep interruptions to remain frequent into toddlerhood for many children. Normal sleeping, waking, and eating habits of newborns do not vary much when you change their feeding methods; because waking is not always about hunger. They have a drive to suckle, partially to encourage milk production. Changing the source of the milk does not totally over-ride their drive. You will have many feeds back-to-back, and many throughout the night. It is developmental when their sleep habits change, and little to do with their food intake.

Infants waking frequently at night is normal and protective. If we view the behavior in the context of our ancestral survival, it has always been beneficial to our survival as a species that infants do this. Sleep and nighttime make us more vulnerable to outside threats, more so than day and awake-times. Parent-infant relationships have evolved from many years of personal survival and species survival inter-relationship building. Thus, babies are driven to connect (and frequently) all night, and their cries stimulate adults to respond, soothe, and protect. This is an especially strong response in the adult that gestated the infant, but extends to other caregivers to a lesser extent, and even lesser but still present in other adults in general.

Babies do sleep for more hours of the day than they are awake, and ranges or averages of normal vary slightly based on the source of data, but in general the ranges are similar. Each child's sleep needs are individual, so just knowing the general expectation can help us to know if there is a problem. Babies less than 2 months old usually sleep 16 to 20 hours a day. Between 3 to 4 months maybe 15 to 18 hours. This sleep is very broken up, so it does not usually seem like they are sleeping a lot, but they are. The first few months it will feel like all they do is sleep or eat, because they do not start really interacting and playing for a few months. They will wake you frequently, day and night. Having interrupted sleep can be particularly challenging for new parents. In fact, interrupting sleep frequently has historically been used as a torture technique in some regions during war-time, just for comparison.

Frequent feeding and waking does not mean they are not getting enough, and they will cluster feed even when their stomach is very full. It also does not mean they are not getting enough sleep. Infant and toddler sleep needs are very different from adult's sleep needs and they do not suffer like we do when they are woken up multiple times per night.

As the baby gets older, they will change their patterns. By 5 months they may be sleeping only 14-15 hours a day. After what many call the four-month sleep regression, they drop about 3 hours of sleep in their 24-hour cycle. This is a time many parents worry about the supply changing, and there is no need. The body will adjust to the baby's new schedule. You might lose some sanity due to the sleep changes, but the changes don't mean baby isn't getting enough to eat.

"Sleep regressions" are named so because it seems that babies go through phases where they sleep very poorly, and the name is meant to reflect that they are regressing in their progress towards a full night of sleep. This is really a misnomer, because they are progressing in other things, which is why they are sleeping poorly. The progress to sleeping through the night is not linear. Sleep regressions are temporary disruptions, and going through them is a normal part of over-all development. For example, when a baby is about to master a new skill or concept their brains are very busy and overstimulated, so their sleeping patterns are disrupted; some call this a "mental-leap". There is often not much to be done for sleep regressions or mental leaps except to ride the wave, wait for it to pass, and find comfort in that it is normal and temporary. Also, take more naps than usual. It is okay to take some pressure off of yourself and cancel your plans for a while when your baby is not sleeping well, it is temporary and you can get back to normal once it's over. Note: these happen to even sleep trained babies, so if you pursue sleep training, you might have to do it more than once after each sleep regression.

The amount of time a baby nurses plays into how much they are sleeping, and it varies quite a bit in the beginning. Feedings may range from 5 to 60 minutes in the first few weeks. Expect to see a suck-swallow-breathe pattern that makes it appear that they are taking a break from nursing for a moment between suckles and swallows. If a lactating person has an extremely fast flow and the baby is very efficient, time at the breast can be 5 to 10 minutes on each side, and then they are done! Some people have slower flows, and some babies are slower to eat so they take maybe 20 to 30 minutes on each breast. Babies also often get a restful light nap while eating and both the feed and the nap, though done simultaneously, still count towards feed time and rest time. Most babies generally become more efficient with time, and tend to have shorter nursing sessions as the months go by. As their required sleep time lessens, they are more likely to stay awake during feeds. If it is unclear to you if the behavior is normal or not, especially after a change, then seek professional assessment and guidance.

As time goes on, babies do eventually sleep in longer stretches. After a few weeks to a few months, once per 24 hours you will get a 4 to 6 hour stretch, but sometimes it takes many months to reach that milestone. Be prepared that some children wake every 2 to 3 hours for years. Yes, I do mean until they are preschoolers. This goes unchanged with changing feeding methods or adding more solids. Because, again, sleep is developmental and unrelated to food intake. It is also biologically appropriate given that our milk content and low capacity is designed for close contact and frequent feeds, versus mammals that have larger capacity and milk content that allows for longer separation so they can leave their young to go hunt. Children and toddlers who are not as reliant on milk should get a solid stretch of 6 plus hours at least once per night, so if this is still not happening by 1-3 years of age you might ask your pediatrician or family practitioner for a sleep study, to see if something fixable is contributing to a lack of adequate rest patterns.

Most infants sleep 12-15 hours a day by 6 to 12 months, but the pattern of solid sleep chunks and length of naps varies greatly. You might have a baby that sleeps two 5-hour stretches at night and takes 2 long 2-hour naps. You might have a baby that sleeps in three 4-hour chunks all night and then takes 2-3 mini-naps a day. Unfortunately, there is no magic formula to predict which pattern you baby will follow. Know that variation is normal!

Most babies sleep through the night by 6 months, but this nugget of information gets misinterpreted often. Sleeping through the night actually means that they give you one solid stretch of 5-6 hours without waking, and spend the other 5-6 hours of sleep waking and eating less frequently than they do during the day. It does not mean they sleep 8-12 hours straight. Additionally, not all babies even do this by 6 months. And it doesn't mean anything is wrong! Most adults do not even go all night without waking to use the restroom or get some water.

Toddlers age 1-2 years average 11-14 hours per 24 hours, and typically still need 1 long nap or 2 short naps during the day. Preschoolers, age 3-5 years sleep around 10-13 hours per day and then typically drop napping or take 1 short nap per day. By school age, most children sleep 9-11 hours per night and do not nap most days. The time spent asleep gets shorter as they get older.

Since most readers are learning about infants, we will return to that age group. We need to start holding babies not only to normal baby standards, but to individualized standards. What is normal for your baby? Are they acting off? Do you have other clues that things are not going well? Can their sleep changes be explained by things like teething, mental leaps, and sleep regressions? If you can't sort out fact from fiction and you are so tired you are cross-eyed, see an IBCLC to assess for lactation issues and your healthcare provider for other potential issues.

When they go through sleep regressions, mental leaps, teething, and developmental milestones those tend to disrupt their sleeping patterns. If it seems you are past all those phases and yet your toddler does not get restful sleep regularly, and is having behavioral issues, they might need evaluation by a sleep or airway specialist to rule out any anatomical or pathophysiological problems that might be causing poor sleep.

You will likely be tempted in your exhaustion to follow a sleep training method, and not all methods are safe or wise in consideration of the lactation relationship, or in consideration of an infant's well-being. That might be why you bought my book. You might also be mistakenly advised by a well-meaning healthcare provider, that does not understand nursing dyad biological norms, that your baby should be sleeping more at their age or for longer stretches. They may advise sleep training or formula, when they should be referring you to an IBCLC to assess if the sleep pattern in relation to the nursing relationship is normal. They do not have all the tips that can help protect lactation yet encourage more rest for the dyad, and that is okay! They are often just sharing things they have heard, but that does not make them the expert on this topic. They also often don't have time or expertise needed to deep dive into troubleshooting this topic with you. This is why we have specialists.

Many ill-informed but well-intentioned people will also often perpetuate a myth that it is bad to let your baby nurse to sleep. This is biologically normal and how they are designed to be comforted into sleeping. The slowing of the milk flow as the breast drains and the surge of feel-good hormones during nursing helps them to relax and lull into a sleeping state. They all eventually fall asleep without the breast, so there is no need to rush stopping this practice; it is not a bad habit. Forcing or pushing babies out of this instinct results in tears on both sides. As your baby gets older, they will start napping without nursing to sleep first, and eventually go to bed without nursing to sleep. You will not find that my suggestions involve putting your baby down and expecting them to fall asleep on their own, which is very unlike most sleep training methods. It is developmentally appropriate for infants to need help falling asleep, as many children and adults do, too. This might not look like nursing to sleep, but it might involve cuddling, rocking, patting, or other physical connection that helps your infant feel safe. People do eventually get in bed and go to sleep without help, and you do not have to force the issue. However, some people will always prefer a cuddle or white noise to help them dose off (like when we shush the baby to sleep).

Sleep training a breastfed baby is so challenging for the modern parent because many sleep consultants ruin lactation relationships, and lactation consultants want you to martyr your sleep to the lactation relationship. It is up to you to find a balance that you can live with. You might have to experiment with how your supply might handle longer stretches of sleep, as this causes some people's supply to dip, or the change cuts out too many feedings per day and causes baby to not get enough overall milk intake. I have seen sleep training take a baby from 8-10 feeds per day to 5 or 6, and because the lactating parent's capacity was only a few ounces at a time that cut out almost half of baby's daily calories. It is important to monitor your baby's diaper counts and weight gain closely if you start forcing the issue of reducing feeds. There is also the chance that if you do not adjust things slowly or carefully enough, you can put yourself at risk of clogs and mastitis. You might have an infant that is sleeping more, but then end up having to wake up to pump. These are also risks when you use machines that promote more sleep, such as mechanical bassinets. This is especially true the younger you pursue altering biologically normal sleep. If you work with a sleep consultant, you should simultaneously work with a lactation consultant to be sure that changes will not affect the baby or lactation negatively.

It is generally safe to encourage, but not force, good sleep habits. Staying on a consistent but flexible schedule for naps and bedtime can encourage good sleep hygiene. For example, go to bed at the same time every night, but be flexible for those nights when baby is calling for a cluster feeding session. Flexibility can reduce frustration for the inevitable interruptions to our typical routines. Another potentially helpful tip is encouraging baby to eat more frequently during the day because it might cut down on the number of typical nighttime feeds, as they meet their needs on a daily basis. Meaning, every 24 hours they accumulate enough intake to meet their growth and function requirements. Additionally, creating a womb-like sleeping space helps baby feel safe and sleep better. This would include having an extremely dark sleep space with a white noise like a fan whirring near the baby. Blocking the windows with contact paper or hanging up blackout curtains might be an option. Sometimes having something that smells like the parents near or in the sleeping space helps. To avoid creating a suffocation hazard, you might wrap a shirt the lactating parent has worn over the cot mattress, if you use one. Warming the baby's bed before laying them in it helps, as well. Form fitting pajamas, swaddling, and sleep sacks help re-create the tight and snuggly feeling of being in the womb. Conversely, you would want a super bright and active atmosphere during the day. Naps can be in brighter rooms to help adjust circadian rhythms of sleep to more light naps during the day, leaving deeper sleep for the night. Noise level can be normal with the hustle and bustle of the house during the day, leaving quieter more restful time during the night hours. These would all encourage good sleep hygiene without interfering with lactation. Of note, swaddling should be stopped within 2 months, and especially once baby can roll over so it is a short-lived aid. Sleep sacks are preferable to swaddling because they allow for more proper hip development, reflex expression, and early feeding cues to be seen. Also, be alert that at 2-3 months of age babies will stop nursing to sleep at every feed during the day, and they will want to stay up and play. This does not mean they are not content, just that they are spending more time awake during the day, and are developmentally ready for more playtime.

Many parents find that nursing and co-sleeping helps to keep them well-balanced. It can also promote more optimal nursing, as parent and baby are able to smell and hear each other all night, and the lactating parent can more closely identify and meet baby's needs. While the AAP recommends avoiding some versions of this, there is evidence contradicting that stance and it goes against the biological norms of the human species for the past tens of thousands of years. Evidence also suggests that risks of co-bedding drop after 3 months of age for non-smoking teetotalers. We will delve more into this in the next section.

As sleep pattern disruption is normal and developmental, you do not necessarily need to do anything different. For example, babies do not need to start eating solids at 4 months because they are waking more, although some people will try to convince you of this; the 4-month sleep regression is developmental and unrelated to solid food intake. When they are very close to mastering a new skill or understanding a more complex concept, they will have a mental leap and they sleep very poorly. This happens as they approach rolling over, crawling, pulling to stand, and walking. It also happens as their mind develops in complexity. They also sleep poorly when they are teething, which happens on and off for years. These are the times you will be tempted to get them to eat more to see if they will sleep better, and it usually will not work.

Babies wake for many reasons other than hunger. They can be seeking connection, be cold, have startled, or been woken by their own bodily functions. Additionally, infants make a lot of very strange noises that do not sound like normal breathing, and they hiccup frequently. They might grunt or groan, or cycle through more rapid breathing episodes. They also might jerk their bodies suddenly while falling asleep or changing positions, or shake their limbs a bit. Being unfamiliar with newborn noises and behaviors often causes parents to needlessly worry. When in doubt, take a video or picture and show it to your healthcare provider to confirm if it is normal or not. Call emergency services if the strange noises are accompanied by rib retractions, or the baby's mouth or face turning blue.

We know that having a responsive caregiver when crying, to signal a need, is critical to mental and emotional health of infants and children. In general, it is beneficial to be responsive to your infant's needs. It teaches them they are safe, and they can trust you. Building upon a parent-child relationship that makes a child feel safe and leads them to trust their caregivers can contribute to raising well-adjusted, independent, and resilient children. It is always okay to do your best to meet their needs and follow your parental instincts. Simultaneously it is also okay to be human and to find the need to change some of the dynamics of the relationship in order to protect your mental and emotional health, too.

Parents also wake or have disrupted sleep for many other reasons than a baby crying and wanting to eat. When we become caretakers of infants our brain changes so that we wake more easily; this change is crucial to our offspring's survival. These changes are more pronounced for parents that carry the infant in pregnancy, though the changes to the brain are apparent in all infant caregivers. Most new female parents also have more sensitive hearing and sleep very lightly. This likely is to the benefit of attending to the baby's needs more readily as well as detecting environmental threats more easily. Another sleep related change for lactating parents of note is the change in ability to be able to sleep on the stomach. Stomach sleepers are often sad to discover that they still have to avoid their favorite sleeping position due to mammae fullness, leaking, needing to avoid clogs, or co-sleeping arrangements. Not sleeping in a favored position can cause us to not feel as well rested. Some parents also have a harder time sleeping when their infant is co-sleeping in the same room, and their frequent waking to every stir of motion is too burdensome to make room-sharing worth it to them.

ORAL TETHERS AND SLEEP

We all have connective tissue under our tongue, lips, and cheeks; sometimes that tissue is too tight, thick, or short, and it keeps the mouth and tongue from moving the way that they should. Tethers can also influence our airway development because the resting tongue posture does not create pressure on the cranial bones in our upper palate. This effects the shape of the nasal airways above it. Airway abnormalities can ultimately cause poor sleep.

Looking further into development ties can continue to impact quality of life and inhibit optimal development. As the facial structures grow tongue tied adults and children often find difficulty with proper breathing, especially when asleep. Common complaints and conditions of tongue-tied people are around heartburn, reflux, snoring, not sleeping well, daytime fatigue, and having poor posture in order to try to breathe well. Children who do not sleep well often exhibit dysfunctional behaviors during the day like poor attention span, destructive tendencies, and crankiness. Tied babies and children often wake more frequently at night than is average.

It is never too late in life to correct the tether with a revision, and in my opinion, it is best to do as soon as the tether is diagnosed. An ounce of prevention is worth a pound of cure! There are more exhaustive lists available online of all the things that oral tethers can effect. This includes nursing, sleep, airway, dentition, orthodontics, jaw tension, neck tension, and much more. The entirety of data around oral tethers would be outside of the scope of this book, but I wanted to highlight its possible effects on sleep. I give a much more extensive explanation on oral tethers in my lactation book, as it is relevant to much more than sleep. There are also much more comprehensive books dedicated to the topic of oral tethers alone. If you are in doubt about oral tethers influencing your baby's sleep (or yours), seek out a professional through the preferred provider network (see Resources).

BREAST-SLEEPING

Many parents find that nursing and co-sleeping helps to keep them well-balanced. It can also promote more optimal nursing as parent and baby are able to smell and hear each other all night, and the lactating parent can more closely identify and meet baby's needs. While some health authorities recommend avoiding this, there is evidence contradicting that stance and it goes against the biological norms of the human species for the past tens of thousands of years. There are also many countries and cultures where breast-sleeping is expected and encouraged. Pretending it is not an option does a disservice to families, so we will explore risks and benefits here.

Breast-sleeping is a term coined by Dr. James McKenna which describes a baby sleeping near a breast all night. He is a Ph. D. in biological anthropology who studies the biological norms and safety of lactating parents and babies sleeping together, while in a nursing relationship. His website and books will answer all your questions about how to breast-sleep safely, and how he collects his data. His information is listed in the "resources" section.

Babies that at least sleep in the same room as their parents tend to nurse throughout the night, and some sleep better with this arrangement. Night nursing is greatly beneficial to over-all supply and infant safety. Babies are designed to desire closeness to their caregiver, so for many babies being in the same room but not the same bed is a good compromise if the parent is not comfortable with bed-sharing. Some parents also choose to bed-share for only part of the night as a compromise. The feeding sessions between 12 and 5 AM are the most crucial to lactation success due to nightly hormonal signaling. It is also when lactating people make the most milk, and thus baby gets the most milk. The frequent wakings are also thought to be protective against Sudden Infant Death Syndrome.

Co-sleeping might be baby in the same room, but it can also mean co-bedding like mentioned above. Even when most parents plan to avoid co-sleeping or co-bedding, they end up doing it anyway or on accident because they are desperate, and sleep deprived. If you have a safety plan, this can help you avoid making risky choices. When you are exhausted you might fall asleep with your baby in an unsafe space. Many suffocation accidents happen when a parent accidentally falls asleep with their infant in recliners and on couches.

The safest space for baby to sleep according to many experts and studies is in their own cot or crib that has a firm mattress, no blankets, no pillows, no stuffed animals, nor bumpers, while lightly and snuggly dressed, and positioned on their back. This has been studied compared to other sleep arrangements and evidence suggests that this carries the lowest risk for babies. In addition, having babies sleeping in the same room the first 6 months of life, but not the same sleep space, reduces risks to babies. Babies do not typically like this arrangement and it triggers their instincts of fear of being alone, they know that being alone is dangerous, and they protest by crying or waking the moment you set them down. It is not a good option for many families, despite it being the safest. The reality is the risk of not doing this drops off significantly after 3 months of age, anyway. The reality is also that you can choose other sleeping arrangements with similar safety outcomes, such as breast-sleeping. Dr. McKenna's research finds that when breast-sleeping, parent and baby sync in heart and breathing rates, both are more physiologically stable when bed sharing, and both get more restful sleep.

That being said, if you are going to sleep with your baby close to you there are some safety tips that should be followed to keep it lower risk, found through Dr. McKenna's research. Both adults that sleep in the bed must be light sleepers and not have taken any drugs or alcohol, including sleep-aids. Even better if it is just the lactating parent and the baby in the bed. Additionally, there should be no blankets or pillows in the bed. The parent and baby should be dressed warmly enough to not need them. Also, the bed should be firm and away from corners or walls, as baby can fall off the bed or fall into a gap and suffocate. Ideally, the bed would be in the middle of a room and the mattress on the floor. Baby's positioning would ideally still be on their back, so the feeding parent should position themself such that they bring the breast to the baby who is positioned safely. Alternatively, you might have the baby laying their back on your arm, while you hold them near your chest. There are many tips and images online on how to most safely co-bed together while nursing, and position adjustments to try. Co-sleeping on the same surface should never be done on soft beds, sofas, or recliners. Dr. McKenna's book and website have the best information, and he conducts his research through the University of Notre Dame. Making the best decisions for your family around sleep are just another challenge of nursing, and parenting.

Additionally, important to note, is that The Academy of Breastfeeding protocol for bedsharing concluded that "evidence does not support the conclusion that bedsharing among breast-feeding infants (i.e., breastsleeping) causes sudden infant death syndrome (SIDS) in the absence of known hazards." Their full statement is available to the public on their website, and I will list that in resources.

Additional international resources will be listed in the "Resource" section from Australia and the UK. Australia's National SIDs council has published through the Red Nose, National Scientific Advisory Group, an Information Statement on sleeping with a baby. The UK has published through Basis, a project of the Durham Infancy and Sleep Centre (DISC), in the Department of Anthropology at Durham University UK, a Baby Sleep Information Source website and app. Both address safe infant sleep under the circumstances of co-sleeping and bed-sharing.

Part of breast-sleeping, as you can imagine, is nursing the

baby to sleep. It is biologically normal for infants to nurse to sleep, and there is no need to avoid doing this. Both the lactating parent and the infant have a surge of hormones that make them sleepy during nursing, so one could argue that it is an intentional part of the larger design to facilitate the rest for both. It is also okay to seek other methods of soothing to sleep to involve other caregivers and give the lactating parent a break, but you should not feel forced to do so. The same is true for nursing toddlers, and sometimes after 1-3 years of night nursing parents decide to night wean because it is making life too difficult. As long as nutritional needs are being met, it is okay to be flexible with nursing to sleep. You will need to consider their nursing needs, temperament, developmental phase, and your own needs.

Babies who breast-sleep also have many feeds where it seems like they are both asleep, yet feeding at the same time. It is true, they are doing both. It is a lighter sleep, more akin to a catnap, but it is still restful and restorative. Sleep cycles for all humans involve going in and out of lighter and deeper cycles.

The most dangerous plan is not having a plan, because when you are sleep deprived to the point of exhaustion you may accidentally fall asleep in an unsafe space with your infant, which is how most accidental infant deaths happen. Martyring yourself to lactation or trying to be a perfect parent is not only unhealthy for the parent but dangerous for the baby. Finding balance and planning for the inevitable exhaustion is a necessity.

Breast-sleeping and co-sleeping are not the answer for all dyads. Some families compromise by spending part of the night breast-sleeping, or using a separate sleep space while still in the same room but still allowing for in-bed feeds. Some babies and some parents sleep horribly when bed-sharing. Some babies nurse more times a night when breast-sleeping, and have a parent that has a hard time falling back asleep once woken. That baby and parent might be happier co-sleeping with a bassinet at the bedside. That baby might be happy to be in its own room, sleeping 6 hour stretches when it can't smell its lactating parent. A parent might decide risks of bed sharing are too high, and opt for another plan.

The variations and nuances are endless. My point being: it's up to you to decide and do your own risk analysis.

An important part of this decision process is evaluating risks, and I especially want to highlight and return to the topic of substance use while bed-sharing. This comes from a place of wanting to inform and educate, not judge.

Because alcohol is so widely used and accepted as a normal part of many people's daily lives, I would like to dedicate a special subsection to discussing alcohol and breast-sleeping.

In general, light alcohol intake is compatible with nursing, but not breast-sleeping. Some health authorities recommend waiting until the baby is 2-3 months old to imbibe, to allow for liver maturity, though some countries and world health authorities disagree that waiting is needed. If you personally feel uncomfortable you can pump your milk and dilute it with other milk later, save it in the freezer for when baby is older, or use it for milk baths. There is never a need to dump milk consumed while having an alcoholic beverage, as the content that goes into the milk is so low. The amount of alcohol in the milk increases and decreases as the amounts in the blood change.

What is more dangerous about alcohol than the content in the milk is the ability to be able to care for the infant when intoxicated. It is best to have a sober caregiver available and avoid doing any co-sleeping on the nights you partake. Of importance is also that alcohol can reduce how efficiently the breast releases milk due to its effects on hormones, and the baby might nurse less due to the flavor changes; so even 1 glass comes with caution. While sometimes beer is reported to help with supply, it can end up having the opposite effect. Alcohol can negatively impact hormones and reduce supply and ability to have letdowns. Of course, the safest option is avoiding alcohol altogether.

On the opposite end of the spectrum of total avoidance of alcohol is the camp that is overly encouraging of utilizing alcohol as a way to cope with the stresses of parenting. There are many people who subscribe to a culture that normalizes and encourages you to indulge to escape, and this can be very dangerous. It is a slippery slope to developing alcoholism when you start using alcohol to cope with the stressful days, because most of the days of early infancy and early childhood are very stressful. This is especially dangerous for parents who are already at risk for developing alcoholism or are suffering from postpartum mood disorders and seeking to self-medicate. Not only does this negatively impact your milk supply, but it can start to affect your parenting.

Even if you avoid the risks of caretaking while under the influence of alcohol and are responsible enough to have a sober caretaker present at all times, alcohol affects your personality when you are sober. The regular consumption of alcohol depletes some vitamins that are key to our neurological, hormonal, and mood stabilization. It is likely to make you feel an exacerbation of the stress that you are trying to avoid and interfere with what could otherwise be quality time with your baby. Alcohol also inhibits the ability of the drinker to get enough deep sleep, so it exacerbates sleep deprivation. Moderate to high alcohol intake can also alter baby's sleep patterns, cause poor weight gain, lead to hypoglycemia, or impair their motor development. There are very good reasons that alcohol is a hot topic. Your baby deserves for you to take a good hard look in the mirror, and at them, to see how you are both affected by the consumption of these drugs, even in moderation. If you are struggling with safe and infrequent consumption, then it might be time to seek help for controlling your alcohol intake.

Other drugs to consider are tobacco, marijuana and illicit or illegal drugs. Smoking, no matter the substance, introduces risks to you and to your baby. Second and third hand smoke expose the baby to toxins, and babies who are around smoke are at high risk for developing asthma, having frequent asthma attacks, having more frequent upper respiratory and ear infections, and have a higher risk of dying from SIDs than babies who are in non-smoking homes. Smoking not only introduces toxins but it alters the nutritional status of the milk. Ideally, no one in the house with a newborn will be smoking inside, and if they smoke outside then they should change clothes and wash their hands when they return. For now, we should assume the same for vaping until proven otherwise.

Drugs can also alter your ability to parent safely and can be passed through your milk to your baby. Some drugs if passed through the milk can result in infant death. Parents that do drugs are often investigated by child protective services, might be separated from their children, and are prohibited from feeding their child breastmilk, even when it is a legal drug in some states, like marijuana. There is not enough evidence to say that nursing and doing any of these drugs is totally and definitely safe, and exposing children to them or causing them to ingest these drugs is illegal in most cases. Ideally, parents will be drug free while caring for their infants and small children. Marijuana is presently a gray area due to evolving legal changes and research developments, but most providers advise avoiding it due to lack of data on its safety during pregnancy and lactation.

If you are struggling with making good choices around drugs and alcohol, I have listed the contact for Substance Abuse and Mental Health Services Administration in my "resources" section, and that is a good place to start. You can also reach out to your healthcare team for help.

Use your best judgement, consult professionals, and error on the side of caution when in doubt.

THE ROLE OF HORMONES

When we are experiencing the sensations of hunger, our body is producing a hormone called ghrelin. Ghrelin is responsible for short term management of food intake, and leptin is responsible for our over-all appetites and long-term regulation. It is possible to get our body in the habit of producing ghrelin on a schedule, based on our typical eating pattern, rather than when our body actually needs to feed. If I train my body to eat 6 meals a day, after a while I am going to get hungry 6 times a day. Conversely, if I start skipping breakfast then eventually my body will stop signaling me to be hungry at breakfast. The ghrelin is mostly produced in anticipation of eating. There is also some ghrelin in breastmilk, likely to encourage the infant to eat frequently. If we as adults do not eat, our body will shut down the hunger signals and use what we have stored in our fat cells until we eat again. If we do this habitually, it will stop signaling us on that schedule and be set on a new pattern of signaling hunger.

So how can we help determine if baby is really truly in need of food or just in a habit of being woken by their hunger hormones? Many infants are able to adjust to eating less at night and then in turn eating more during the day, and they stay on projected and healthy growth patterns. In fact, over time, this is what all infants do. Now, this says nothing of when infants wake to nurse because they are seeking something other than food. They also nurse for thirst, comfort, and connection. They might wake up because they are cold, wet, need to burp, or are seeking physical connection. Babies are wired to need human touch, and they recognize that being alone is dangerous and scary. They do not wake only to eat, but it is likely at least some of the time that some of their wakings are due to spikes in ghrelin.

If you are struggling with the thought of withholding or delaying nursing, it's okay to rethink your plans around sleep training. Continue to evaluate and re-evaluate. Ask yourself: Is my need and our goal worth some temporary stress? Babies go through many stressful phases like teething and sleep pattern disruption when approaching milestones. It is ok to decide that your need for more adequate rest outweighs your desire to avoid any stressors for your baby. Only you can answer what you need, and what methods you are comfortable using to meet those needs. It is up to you to do your own risk-analysis, I am just here to present information and options.

Hormones in milk and milk production also play a role in timing and frequency of feeding, as well as regulating sleep patterns. Understanding this can help you understand my methodology and suggestions, so I will expand on that some.

Morning milk tends to have more volume, and less fat. Babies need to hydrate in the morning after going long stretches without drinking. Night milk tends to have less volume but more fat, and the higher fat in a full belly allows for greater satiety and longer stretches between feeds. Depending on the time of day the milk will have different levels of hormones and other particles to encourage baby to be awake or to sleep, such as melatonin. It is available in the milk to work with baby's natural hormone rhythms to encourage sleep and wake cycles.

The concentration is not enough to over-power the natural patterns so do not worry too much about keeping track of what time you pumped your milk, if you are feeding pumped milk. Parents who do not track time pumped versus time fed do not experience a higher incidence of sleep issues in their infants. It does not hurt to track this and try to match these up, especially if you are struggling with getting to a normal sleep and wake pattern. It is not something to obsess over, just keep an eye on.

Milk production is largely driven by the hormone prolactin. It starts with the delivery of the placenta causing a huge drop in progesterone, which is needed in order to have the huge spike in prolactin, which leads to the milk coming in. Milk supply is then built upon based on frequent prolactin spikes, caused by breast stimulation and milk-gland drainage, and the subsequent hormonal feedback loop that happens with those actions. The circadian rhythm of prolactin is such that it boosts from 12 to 5 AM and bottoms out in the early evening, and thus the milk supply is higher from midnight to noon than it is from noon to midnight. So, for example, the mammae might make 4 to 5 ounces in the nighttime and early morning feeds but make only 2 to 3 ounces in the early evening feeds. The 12 to 5 am prolactin boost is important for 2 reasons: higher milk volume and setting your over-all prolactin course for the next 24-72 hours. Cluster feeding may happen between midnight and five in the morning due to the abundance of milk flow and baby's instincts to night-feed, some babies get 20% of their daily intake during this time frame. This not only helps them get large volumes of milk but it also serves to stimulate the daily prolactin amounts, and thus overall daily milk production. When you do not get stimulation during the critical prolactin peak the first year of nursing then your supply will most likely drop off, and sometimes even dry up.

There is a real and serious risk of supply reduction and early weaning if you remove too many night feedings, or remove feedings during the critical prolactin boost time frame. This is not to say that feeding less frequently at night poses the same risk, but close monitoring and realistic expectations are essential if you plan to continue to lactate. It is unlikely that any method that aims to get your child to sleep for 7 or more hours per night or suggests you skip feeds from 12 am to 5 am is compatible with a long term lactation relationship. The longer the stretch of sleep for some one with a low capacity, the riskier it is. This is due to the feedback inhibition hormones that are produced with a full breast. Feedback Inhibitor of Lactation is produced in higher quantities the more time that is spent with a full breast, and having too much of this feedback can cause supply decrease or supply to dry up. This poses a secondary risk of your infant refusing to nurse due to the lack of volume they are accustomed to, which can further push the issue of weaning due to lack of nursing. Many sleep training methods are associated with early weaning. Allowing for no more than 1 stretch of 6 hours of rest per 24 hours helps mitigate this risk for most people, with the other night feeding spacing remaining every 2-4 hours. Some have a high enough capacity that two 6 hour stretches are tolerated long term.

Sleep on formula versus breastmilk is another thing to consider when making your choices about feeding and sleep, especially as I am sure you have heard many myths around this. Formula is harder for babies to digest and so some babies tend to sleep maybe 3 to 4 hours at a time after a formula bottle rather than the typical 2 to 3 hours after breastmilk, and they seem to sleep more deeply. Many parents notice that if they give a formula bottle at night versus breastmilk, they get a longer stretch of sleep. As tempting as that is to do for night feeds, it is actually over-riding protective benefits of nursing and waking frequently. It also over-rides the baby's instincts to build and protect the milk supply. When a baby human feeds frequently and wakes frequently at night this is protective against Sudden Infant Death Syndrome (SIDS), and is protective to the lactation relationship. Additionally, babies who get all or mostly formula tend to sleep more at night because they are meeting all their intake needs during the day with large bottles. Formula fed infants often feed twice as much per feed versus their breastfed counterparts, which means they are less driven at night to wake to meet intake needs. It is logistically easier for a formula feeding parent to sleep train, because they do not have to consider lactation needs as part of their risk analysis and plan of action. If you are having to or choosing to give formula, it is best to try to also provide some breast milk to help balance the risks to lactation and continue to provide the protective benefits of the breastmilk. If you incorporate formula into your nighttime routine, I would suggest alternating with nursing and avoiding going more than 4-6 hours once per night without nursing or pumping until at least 6 months postpartum.

After the supply is more established, some parents can get away with going two long stretches without hampering overall supply. For some people with low supply and low capacity, they need to maintain nursing or pumping every 2-3 hours for 9-12 months in order to maintain lactation. For many parents it requires being over 1 year postpartum for the supply to be established well enough and not as hormonally driven in order for that plan to work while still being able to nurse. However, by then many babies are sleeping in longer stretches regardless.

COMBINING IT ALL TO MAKE A PLAN

First, I want to say this: you don't have to sleep train. There is no universal law or plan that works for every baby, or for every parent, or for every family. Many parents do different things for each child depending on that child's sleep patterns, nursing patterns, and habits. Sleep training is not a rite of passage. All babies eventually sleep longer stretches, and independently. Parents make different decisions based on if the current situation is working or not. Parents might make changes depending on when naps can be caught more easily or not. Parents make decisions that work at the time for a multitude of reasons. Maybe you read everything I have had to say so far, and you have decided not to sleep train after all. Or maybe you have decided to wait it out a few months. Maybe you just want to sleep train partially, to get a longer stretch of sleep part of the night. Maybe you try this out a few nights and abandon it. Each family must do their own risk analysis, prioritize what is important to them, and accept the risks of their decisions. Regardless of what you decide, know that I am here to support you. I want you to trust your instincts and make decisions for yourself. Before getting into my suggestions to help extend sleep cycles, I want to talk about how to get more rest in general.

To facilitate rest for a lactating parent, it is important to note that most lactating people can go up to 6 hours without nursing or pumping once in a 24 hour period without it dramatically impacting daily supply. Many parents like to take advantage of this by incorporating pumping and bottle feeding into their routine. The baby will likely still want or need to eat in that resting time, so a partner can give the baby pumped milk when it cues. Your lactation consultant can teach you alternate ways of feeding if you feel strongly about avoiding bottles. To replace the missed stimulation, the lactating person can pump an extra time early in the morning when they are most full due to higher prolactin, and take their turn resting in the early evening when it is at its lowest. That way the mammae might allow for the rest without waking them in pain from fullness, and they miss the pump and feeding sessions when output is the lowest. This also allows for a person to keep the same number of mammae stimulating and draining sessions per 24 hours, and reach the typical goal of 8-12 feeding or pumping sessions per 24 hours. Sessions do not have to be a nice, neat every 2-3 hours and can be done with some sessions being back to back, much like how babies cluster feed. Your ability to meet your daily output goal for milk depends on your mammae storage capacity, and frequent draining, for the first year of lactation. If you are happy to use supplemental milk like formula, it is ok to risk this and be flexible in your rest and feeding routine. You might have to experiment with how your supply might handle longer stretches of sleep, as this causes some people's supply to dip, or the change cuts out too many feedings per day and causes baby to not get enough overall milk intake. There is also always the risk of bottle preference (especially without paced-feeding), nursing strikes, and supply dipping when you use bottles as part of your routine—it is up to you to decide if that risk is worth it, no one else. Tips on paced-feeding are readily accessible online and should be reviewed with whomever is to offer the bottle. If preference occurs, these things can usually be overcome with patience and skill, and while it is a risk—it is not a guaranteed outcome.

Having a realistic plan is so important because a high risk factor for postpartum mood disorders, especially postpartum psychosis, is lack of sleep. Prioritizing sleep is so important, and often not given enough attention or consideration when planning for the time frame when new parents are in the throes of newborn life. If you do not set yourself up to get some sleep, you will actually have a harder time falling asleep the more over-tired you are. Work with your healthcare team and the people who are living with you to make a safe sleep-plan. If you find that you are unable to sleep, you need to tell your healthcare provider. What I list here are some options to consider to facilitate better rest, but they may not work out for you.

You might find you need to change the scene in order to get adequate rest. Some parents have better rest if they use ear plugs, play white noise, or have the baby at a different location entirely. If you have a safe way for someone else to take care of the baby for a good 6 hour stretch, you might be able to safely take a low dose sleeping aid, herbal or pharmaceutical. Not every parent wants to be with their baby 24/7 the first few years of their life, so it is ok to admit if you need a break, especially if it is to rest. Most people's supply would likely tolerate a weekly longer stretch of rest, for 6-8 hours, and then be able to rebound over the next few days. Sometimes just knowing the baby is safe with family or friends is enough to allow for a deeper and more adequate rest. Using pharmacological or herbal sleeping aids would best be discussed with your healthcare provider to assure all appropriate safety measures and precautions were covered and in place. You would also need to avoid these if breast-sleeping. Infant Risk organization is also a great resource for finding out if an option is safe (see Resources section).

When your baby is gaining well, your supply is established, and you have an idea of how much milk you make, what your breast capacity is, what size feeds your baby prefers, how many times per 24 hours your baby eats, and what your baby's growth trajectory is, you can start adjusting things. The least risky time to try to change sleep habits is after an infant is 1 year of age. The younger you attempt this, the greater the challenges and risks. My methods and suggestions will only be to encourage 1-2 longer stretches of sleep at night, likely in 3-6 hour stretches, as most lactating people's milk supply cannot tolerate a 7-12 hour stretch every night, at least not without significantly reducing supply, causing more frequent clogs and mastitis, or increasing the risk of totally drying up the supply. It might introduce some risk of clogs but an infrequent rest of that length could probably be recovered from, maybe 2-4 times per month. If you are looking for a 7-12 hour stretch of sleep every night while simultaneously keeping a nursing or lactation relationship going, it is just not a realistic goal before 1 year postpartum. After 1 year supply is less dependent on nightly prolactin stimulation, and that long of a stretch of rest would be a more realistic goal for an infant over 12 months of age.

Utilizing all of the information we have reviewed, plus the hormonal hunger signal patterns that your baby's body has established, you begin the bio-hack of the lactation relationship. Of note, this is only a helpful technique to extend sleep cycles if your child is waking due to hunger signals, this does not include waking due to a wet diaper, feeling cold, wanting connection, or other reasons. Some babies will wake frequently regardless of hunger signals.

The general plan I suggest is that you will slowly push out the time that your baby's body signals them to wake to eat. I do not suggest attempting to adjust more than one feeding session at a time, to avoid over-stressing the parent and infant. When you are pushing-out a feed you do it very gradually, and continue to comfort your infant in other ways, and engage in other distracting behaviors while waiting to begin the feed. This means rocking, cuddling, swaying, shushing, changing, walking around, talking, offering a pacifier, and any other comfort techniques you find helpful. Some parents also find offering a 1-2 ounce bottle of warm water for babies over 6 months helpful to extend feed times while keeping baby comforted and distracted. Pacifiers and small bottles of water are particularly helpful because suckling is very soothing to the nervous system.

I do not recommend you leave the baby alone nor should you expect the baby to self-soothe. They need reassurance and comforting through these changes. The crying is not what is harmful to them, but rather crying without an attempt to be comforted. Leaving babies alone to cry is usually too stressful to the parent, and to the baby. This just isn't necessary when there are other ways to achieve your goals.

Gradual spacing of the feed in this scenario means changing the routine in about 5 minute increments every 3-7 days. This length of time should be enough to slowly shift the ghrelin signaling patterns every week or so. I will walk through some examples with details, so you can mentally walk through all the details to consider.

Feedback on if the plan is going well will center around diaper output and weight gain. Diapers should be monitored daily to assess for adequate urine output and no major changes to bowel habits, and weight should be checked at 1-4 week intervals. Adequate urine output usually indicates adequate hydration. Regular bowel habits and good weight gain indicate adequate nutritional intake. Check weight every 1-2 weeks if there is any question or doubt of baby not getting enough intake. This would also be a helpful interval if you think you might need to recover your milk supply from a change that might lower it. A 3-4 week interval for weight checks would be fine if you feel reassured that the transition is going smoothly.

I will mention here, after giving some background information my opinion is that it is best to wait for supply establishment, a some-what predictable eating schedule, and development of a trusting relationship between the dyad before attempting any sleep training methods or sleep adjusting programs, so at a minimum 4-6 months. Many babies are still regularly waking extra on some nights for growth spurts in the first 4-6 months, and this does still happen after that but much less often. In an ideal world I would not recommend any manipulation of sleep before 1 year of age due to developmental changes of the baby, as well as logistics of the milk supply; but, I know this is not realistic or feasible for some families. It is very important that you are sure that your baby's hunger and thirst needs are met every day, so they should have an abundance of wet and soiled diapers, as well as healthy weight gain and other growth trajectories.

The younger you try any method, the greater the risk of

interrupting lactation and having to re-do the process multiple times throughout the upcoming months when the baby has milestones, growth spurts, or is teething. Sleep-training or trying to extend sleep cycles does not always work and it definitely does not always stick long-term. You might try this method for a week and have a baby that is just not having it. We can make all the plans in the world with all of the best intentions, but your baby is a whole separate person that needs consideration and respect. If the overall signal from the baby is that they cannot tolerate this adjustment, then go back to the drawing board. Ok now, we can get into some examples of ways we might try to manipulate sleep and hunger hormones to get longer sleep cycles.

Example 1:

Say we have a 6 month old infant on the 30th percentile, he has always had excellent diaper output and stayed on his growth curve patterns. His breastfeeding parent's capacity when she is most full is estimated to be around 10 ounces per session, which they notice at their morning pumping sessions when they are most full. The baby often takes 1 breast and the other always gets 5 ounces out, no matter what. She is also able to pump 10 ounces total, if her baby occasionally sleeps through his 5 am feeding. The estimate of what baby typically drinks is about 3-5 ounces per sitting, and he eats 8 times in 24 hours. This has been estimated based on several weighted feeds. He is a predictable baby, and eats every 3 hours on the dot. This pattern is starting to exhaust his parents, especially now that his lactating parent is back at work and naps are harder to come by.

His parent wants to try to get a longer stretch of sleep in the early evening, avoiding disrupting the 12-5 am feeds, to avoid changing her overall daily milk output. He usually eats at 7 pm, and sleeps until 10 pm, when he wakes to eat again. His next feed is usually around 1 am. She will begin the process by going to comfort him but avoiding nursing him immediately. She chooses the 10 pm time because it is most predictable, it is usually a very short feed, and it avoids disrupting the hormone signals between

12 am and 5 am that affect her over-all daily supply total. It is also a low risk time to choose because of the relative lower supply at this time; she is less likely to develop clogs if she pushes out this feeding.

She will wait 5 minutes longer than usual, for 3 to 6 nights in a row. The new feed time is 10:05 pm. She still rocks, changes, shushes, cuddles, and loves on her baby, so he knows he is safe and loved. His crying indicates his hunger signals have woken him up and he wants to eat. In the event it is security and attachment that he is seeking, and not food, then she provides that in other ways. After his initial cries of waking, he settles back down with her comforting techniques. You could choose to employ tools like a pacifier or offering a small bottle of warm water at this point, but this parent did not end up needing to. Infants 6 to 12 months of age are allowed 2 to 4 ounces of water per day.

After the 3 to 6 nights, when the baby starts waking a few minutes later, she waits another 5 minutes out, so 10 minutes from the original wake time. For another 3 to 6 nights she stays at a 10 minute hold, not nursing until 10:10 pm. Now you might imagine that this stretches the time between waking and feeding to 10 minutes, but it usually doesn't. The baby actually starts waking up later by night 6, closer to 10:10 pm. The ghrelin hormones that make the stomach start signaling the brain have adjusted. The time from wake to feed should still be about 5 minutes, it is just 5 minutes later than the few days before. If the baby resists this change after a week, it would be best not to force the issue.

After that, she waits until 10:15 pm. After another 3 to 6 nights until 10:20 pm, and so on and so forth. Eventually, the feed is dropped or pushed back to 6 hours later. For some babies this takes slowly pushing it out over time, and for some after about an hour of pushing it out they just drop the feed entirely. Instead of feeding at 7 pm, 10 pm, and 1 am the baby now eats at 7 pm, and 1 am. The baby's body will no longer wake him at 10 pm by flooding him with the hunger hormones, because it no longer expects to be fed at that time. He might still wake to eat in the window from 7pm to 1 am later down the road if he has a growth spurt, mental leap, or is teething, but his new normal most nights will be to sleep a 6 hour stretch.

After 1 month on this new regimen, his growth is assessed. He is still on track. The lactating parent's capacity and daily overall milk production has slightly decreased, as is noted by mostly 6 to 8-ounce pumps in the morning when he occasionally sleeps through his 4 am feed, rather than 10 ounces she was getting previously; or if she pumps the opposite side of nursing she gets 3-4 ounces. Her typical pump output while at work is unaltered. It seems she is still making plenty for this baby's needs. His lactating parent is better rested, and now more willing to continue the breastfeeding relationship.

The parent repeats the pattern at the 1 am feed when the baby is around 8 months old, assessing if she can avoid disrupting her daily capacity. The new nighttime feeding times are 7 pm and 4 am, so the baby gets a 9 hour stretch of sleep. She now has to pump or hand express around 9 pm most nights to avoid getting uncomfortably full at night, and avoid clogs. However, this gets her a couple of hours in the evening alone followed by a 7 hour stretch of rest most nights. His parents monitor his daily diaper count, and there is no change. Growth of the baby is evaluated after 1 month based on his weight, and is still on track. The baby also now has introduced solids, and is progressing well developmentally.

After a couple of months, when the baby is about 10 months old, the parent attempts to drop the 4 am feed, and when this is done weight gain falls off track at a 2 week follow up, and overall supply decreases dramatically. They do a 2 week weight check rather than 1 month due to the baby acting frustrated at the breast and pump output overall being about 30% lower when she pumps on work days, despite troubleshooting all possible contributors to pump output decrease. For this parent, the bio-hack of the lactation relationship that works for now allows at maximum a 7-9 hour stretch at night, at this stage postpartum. Re-introducing the 4 am feeding resolves all issues within 1 week. The mother and baby have reached a point where they are both happy and thriving, and they had some room to experiment. This can be re-evaluated again when the baby is over 1 year postpartum and the milk production logistics change. This might not have worked out similarly for a mother with a smaller capacity.

Example 2:

This baby is 7 months old, and nursing every 2-3 hours with one 5 hour stretch at night. The parent's estimated per feed capacity is about 3-4 ounces, and her daily supply is high, as well as her refill-rate. If she feeds or pumps every 2-3 hours she can get 36 ounces per day, which she has done when separated for work trips. She otherwise works from home most days. Her baby usually nurses to sleep at around 6 pm, and wakes again at 8 pm, 10 pm, 12 am, 5 am, and 7 am. He does give her that lovely 5 hour stretch every night, but she is exhausted from feeding every 2 hours the rest of the night. During the day he is more distracted and usually eats every 3 hours, at around 10 am, 1 pm, 4 pm, and then 6 pm. He eats 9 times in 24 hours, so she estimates that he gets about 27-30 ounces per 24 hours. This is enough to sustain him on the 50th percentile growth curve, and he is otherwise well hydrated and content. Several weighted feeds done at her IBCLC's office have shown he takes about 3 ounces per feed, sometimes a bit more in earlier morning feeds. Following the bio-hack routine, she slowly stretches out the 10 pm feed (because this is typically a very short nursing session) and eventually he drops the feed. He now eats around 6 pm, 8 pm, 12 am, 5 am, and 7 am throughout the night and early morning. This gives her a 4-hour and 5-hour stretch to rest, which she finds much more sustainable.

One thing this family chose to do differently is that the feeding time is extended by the partner going in and comforting the baby for 5 minutes every night for about a week (rather than 3 to 6 days), and then pushing back by 5 minutes every week thereafter. He eventually drops the 10 pm feed, altogether. The baby seems to make up for this loss by eating more frequently in the early morning. Rather than waiting until 10 am to eat, he eats at 9 am. His other daytime feeds adjust slightly and are now around 9 am,

12 pm, 3 pm, and 6 pm. He still feeds 8 times in 24 hours, and his new intake estimate is roughly 24-27 ounces per 24 hours. Since she is awake and with him, this daytime adjustment is a fair trade off for his parent. She has utilized bio-hacking successfully for her specific circumstance, and her capacity and high refill rate allows for the schedule change. As baby takes more to solids, he stretches out his daytime feeds such that he eventually nurses 6 times in 24 hours by around 10 months. She is unable to drop below 6 feeds per 24 hours without his weight and her supply being affected, so for now this is the most sleep she can work in, in a few months they can re-evaluate.

Example 3:
This dyad is around 4 months postpartum, and the Mom's estimated per feed capacity is around 2-2.5 ounces. This is based solely on weighted feeds, as Mom does not pump at all. The baby eats every 2-2.5 hours around the clock to get around 24-30 ounces per day. This baby has great growth at this rate, but mom is just worn out. She kept waiting for feedings to space out, but they never did. She does not consider this a sustainable lactation relationship. She uses the bio-hack technique to cut out her 9 pm feed, and her baby falls off her growth curve significantly when they compare her 5 month and 6 month weight checks. She and her partner talk it over and decide to introduce formula to over-come this. They introduce a bottle of formula a few hours after her last nursing session of the night, but her partner gives it, and she does not add a pumping session. Rather, they choose to pri-oritize mom's rest and the longevity of the nursing relationship over exclusively giving breastmilk. They keep the bottle size 2.5 ounces so it is similar to the quantity of milk she typically gets. On the infrequent nights that she seems to want more, Mom wakes to feed her to help maintain the balance of combo feeding. They have the baby weighed again after 2 weeks on the new routine and she is gaining adequately again. This gives mom a 4-5 hour stretch of rest at night. She is now more physically and mentally able to maintain her nursing relationship, and is better rested. She

and her partner are fine with combo feeding, the baby gets 1 bottle of formula per day and nurses the rest of the time and from that point forward stays on her growth curve. Her over-all supply does not seem to be negatively impacted drastically. Her goal of nursing 1 year seems more attainable, and the whole family is happy with the change.

After another couple of months they want to try to add another formula bottle at night, and in order to do this without interfering with supply they wait until the 5 am feed to do so. This changes the schedule at night to look like a 7 pm feed at the breast, 9 pm bottle, 12 am breast session, 3 am breast session, a 5 am bottle, and 7 or 8 am nursing session. This gives mom two stretches throughout the night of 4-5 hours while allowing for frequent stimulation during the critical prolactin peak timeframe. She also decides to start breast-sleeping during this stretch from 11 pm to 5 am, and this helps her feel more rested. This dyad has also utilized bio-hacking of the lactation relationship successfully, it just looks slightly different than expected.

ADDITIONAL TIPS TO GET MORE REST

You might ultimately decide, this method doesn't work for you and your family, and that is okay! Maybe it isn't the right time, or the stress of it is too much. I have other tips that I will offer here about how to get more rest.

My greatest suggestions to combat sleep deprivation are to: manage your expectations, take turns feeding at night in two separate 6-hour shifts if you have anyone at all available to help, and take a lot of naps. Get naps however you can. Take family and friends up on watching the baby while you catch a nap, hire a babysitter just so you can nap, or put the baby somewhere safe like a play pen and catch a nap while they watch their mobile or kick their kicky pad.

My other main suggestion is to habitually go to sleep about 3 to 4 hours before you normally would, pre-baby. You will no longer get 6 to 8 hours of solid sleep, as it will now be very interrupted. A good 9-12 hours of scattered and interrupted sleep feels a bit more restful than 8 hours of interrupted sleep.

We should utilize modern technology to our advantage, so if you can catch a longer stretch somewhere by pumping once a day and giving one bottle a night then go for it. If you do not have a partner to help, enlist the help of another family member or a night nanny if you can. Utilize supplemental milk if it means it helps your mental health and helps you reach your lactation goals.

Babies often like to be held while they are napping, so sometimes it is in vain to fight that. Other than wearing your baby it also helps to have other people around to take turns holding them, if possible. Babies napping on your chest is a common way to comfort your baby as well as let them get better sleep, and they like to hear your heart-beat. You will need to be awake when they do this to monitor them, but it is not a problem and is normal for them to want to do this. It does not spoil them but teaches them that they can trust you and that they have a loving, nurturing, and responsive caregiver. Consistently meeting your baby's needs fosters independence because it helps them feel secure and safe. So, they do eventually outgrow this desire and start sleeping well in their own sleeping space. Additionally, sleep begets sleep. Babies that get enough quality nap time during the day sleep better at night.

You can try to adjust everyone's sleep schedule to the baby, even if that means everyone goes to bed at 7 pm, because that is when baby sleeps the longest. A "family bedtime" is a great way to get everyone to bed and then sneak away for a few hours of alone time, or couples time. Additionally, implementing a "family nap time" where everyone in the house takes a midday nap when the baby does can also help keep everyone well rested. Older children might just have to lay quietly in a safe and confined space, such as on a nap mat next to your bed. You can offer them quiet activities to do. If you are not opposed, you could offer a tablet with a headset to keep them occupied with some games or shows for entertainment.

Make sleep, and not chores, a priority. It is okay; everyone with a newborn has a house that looks like a tornado came through it. Sleep when the baby sleeps is only an annoying motto if you choose to not take it as a serious suggestion, and choose not to let go of a few things. Parenthood is usually humbling in this way, and many other humbling experiences are to follow. If you cannot sleep when the baby sleeps, at least rest while the baby sleeps. Outsource as much as possible, and learn to accept the chaos for a while. When you are further along in your healing process postpartum you won't crave as much rest, and the energy for other tasks will return.

In fact, make sleep your top priority for a while. Choose staying on consistent sleep schedules over errands and outings. Still make time for them, but choose sleep first. Be flexible of course, because things happen. However, a consistent pattern of resting at the same times every day helps establish good sleep habits. This might also help give you insight into planning activities around sleep times. This is hard to do with infants under 4 months, and easier following the 4 month sleep regression.

Take the opportunity to make positive sleep associations other than nursing, because this will help others get the baby to sleep when you are unavailable or need a break. This would include rocking, cuddling, playing certain songs, associating sleep with certain smells, patting their booty gently, using white noise, or any soothing activities you choose.

As time goes on, babies do eventually sleep in longer stretches. After a few weeks, once per 24 hours you will get a 4 to 6 hour stretch; but sometimes it takes a few months to reach that milestone. Know that frequent feeding is normal, biologically beneficial, and crucial to maintaining a lactation relationship. Be prepared that some children wake every 2 to 3 hours for years. Sometimes just having realistic expectations takes a lot of the stress out of the situation.

Remember, your child will sleep through the night without needing you... eventually.

MYTHS ABOUT NURSING, FOOD, AND SLEEP

Another consideration that often comes up around night nursing is the health of the teeth. There is no solid evidence that links night nursing to tooth decay, and breastfeeding can be protective against oral health issues. You can further reduce risks by having good oral hygiene. Tooth decay is often due to hereditary issues, poor oral hygiene, too many sugars in the solid diet, oral tethers, and imbalanced oral bacterial flora. There is no reason to avoid nursing at night after teeth have erupted, but there might be issues with bottles. While the bottle may contain breastmilk, the issues are around the mechanics. When bottles are left with the baby, they might fall asleep with it in their mouth and then the milk is pooling in the mouth rather than being swallowed. Pooling can also happen around lip ties, leading to caries on the top 4 front teeth. When feeding on a breast the milk is aimed at the back of the mouth, passed the teeth, and then swallowed. Pooling of milk around teeth happens less often when fed on the breast versus with a bottle. Best practice is not to leave the bottle with the baby in their sleep space, and to stop bottles at 12-18 months of age.

This brings us to our topic of introducing solids! It is a very exciting time, and many try to rush to it. It can even be a relief for a lactating parent to not be the only source of nutrition for baby. You have a lot to consider when starting solids, like when and what to feed! The most recent literature suggests that sometime between 4 to 6 months most children are ready to start solids. I believe the body does not lie and their little bodies tell us when they are ready. As I mentioned before, the sleep regression at 4 months is often mistaken as a sign of readiness, but it is not. Babies' bodies signal they are ready for solids when they lose their tongue thrust reflex, they are able to sit up without assistance, and they have developed a pincher grasp. These changes happen, coincidentally, between 4-6 months.

The tongue thrust reflex is what helps them draw the breast deep into the mouth. If you tickle their mouth or chin, they should thrust their tongue out. This is often mistaken as a sign of hunger when caregivers touch their mouth and the baby sticks their tongue out, but they cannot help but exhibit this reflex when prompted. They are less likely to respond to the reflex when in a deep sleep or when they are very full. It is much like the reflex in your knee that causes your leg to move when the doctor hits below your knee just right. If they are tongue thrusting without being tickled, they are probably actually hungry. In order to draw food into the mouth and not just thrust it out and waste it, that reflex must stop happening. This reflex naturally goes away between 4 to 6 months.

Being able to sit up without assistance is important as it demonstrates that the baby has the core strength needed to attempt to cough out food if they gag or start to choke on it. Again, for most babies this strength develops between 4-6 months of age. They need plenty of opportunity to practice sitting up so they can develop the strength in their muscles. The sitting needs to happen without an aid, like an infant chair.

Finally, having developed a pincher grasp allows them to pinch and grab the food, and practice their hand-eye coordination by bringing the food to their mouth. Their body showing this sign of readiness is an important clue, just as the others are.

All of these signs should be present before offering solids, and you will also often see babies start reaching for food or staring at people who are eating around this time. Food before one is not just for fun, as is often touted; it is important for development.

However, the volume of food actually swallowed does not need to be very much, as breastmilk or formula is their main source of nutrition for the first year. Solid food offered between 4 and 12 months is for developmental milestones, practice with hand eye coordination, practicing chewing and swallowing, and is an introduction to different flavors and textures. They need practice with handling, chewing, and swallowing foods to be able to successfully eat well after age one. It also helps prevent the development of food allergies when you introduce foods before one year of age. The most recent evidence suggests we should introduce high allergen foods to babies before their first birthday to help prevent allergy development.

This is also around the time that you can start offering water. Babies should not get water before solids are started due to the danger it poses to their organs. Formula and breastmilk contain enough hydration and the right balance of electrolytes. This is also why properly mixing formula is so important. Small amounts of water with solids are okay, and might help prevent constipation. The AAP suggests around 4 to 8 ounces of water per day are okay between 6 to 12 months of age, so you can try offering 1-2 ounces each time you offer solids. This will also help with practicing to use cups and straws, as the excitement of a new drink will encourage them to work towards using those items. Other conservative and less risky estimates are that 2 to 4 ounces of water per day is safe, to avoid replacing the nutrient dense breastmilk or formula with too much water intake.

There are a few safety rules with introducing solids I want to cover briefly. It is suggested to avoid letting babies taste honey the first year, as their immune system is not ready to kill or destroy the botulism spores that might be present. This is true even of cooked honey, as heat does not destroy the spores. The only drink you need to avoid is any milk that is not formula or breastmilk. Dairy products can be introduced, such as cheese and yogurt. However, other milks should not replace breastmilk or formula before they are 1 year old, as other milks do not have proper salt and fat content, which puts their kidneys and brain development at risk. Even after 1 year, most non-animal milk substitutes do not have enough fat to be a good replacement. Rather than seeking to replace milk, you can just aim for healthy fat foods in the diet, like fish, eggs, avocado and nut butters. Nut butters are safer if you thin the consistency to avoid a choking hazard. It is also good practice to avoid sugary drinks like soda and juice, due to their connection to poor oral health and chronic disease development. Additionally, choking hazard foods need to be cut into smaller, longer, thinner pieces, or avoided altogether if that is not possible (like popcorn).

SLEEP AIDS OR SLEEP CRUTCHES

Pacifiers

How can we talk about infant sleep without talking about pacifiers? The main concerns with regards to lactation are that there will be nipple confusion, and you might miss feeding cues. Every time a baby is suckling on a pacifier that is a missed opportunity to be suckling and draining the mammae, building supply and connection. You should be safe if you use discretion with pacifiers. Give it after or between feeds or when you need a moment to prepare to feed, and do not ignore the need to cluster feed. Your baby has a strong desire to suckle frequently, and this works in tandem with your mammae needing to have frequent stimulation, so it is not a suitable substitute for the teat more than sparingly a few times a day for the first few weeks. Examples of appropriate times to use it briefly might be while you are driving, during medical procedures, or if the lactating parent is held up momentarily in the shower or going to the restroom. Many babies do well without ever having had one, and using one is mostly just a parenting choice. There is less risk with pacifier use once the supply and demand of nursing is more established in an older infant.

Often, I find parents and professionals want to blame the pacifier for "nipple confusion" because the baby stops latching well, and usually this is a quick and effortless way to avoid thoroughly investigating why the baby will not latch. It is usually not the pacifier's fault, and it is because the baby is unhappy at the breast due to lack of flow or lack of ability to draw out milk. A parent often uses the pacifier because the baby is eating non-stop, and then this happens to coincide with when the baby starts refusing the breast due to lack of flow. If your baby is refusing your breast you need an IBCLC's help, not to avoid pacifiers. Short term judicious use might be indicated, and sometimes pacifiers are used in suck-training therapy to help babies strengthen the muscles they use to breastfeed. The most recent systematic analysis of pacifier use by the World Health Organization in 2016 found that there was not a statistically significant difference in breastfeeding success at 3 months postpartum for dyads that used pacifiers from the first few days on, versus those that did not. Studies have also shown that pacifier use reduces the risk of SIDs.

You also want to consider the pacifiers effect on oral health, dental health, and speech. When you do not wean a baby off of a pacifier by 1 year, you risk issues in these developments. Sucking on bottles and pacifiers should ideally stop around one year, so that the child can learn to use their oral muscles properly, and their palate and teeth are not molded into problematic forms. It is also more challenging to convince a toddler to give up a pacifier, than an infant. Also, keep in mind using a pacifier sets you up to have to fetch it frequently when it falls out of your baby's mouth, sometimes several times a night during sleeping times. While they can be a helpful tool, they do have their down-sides. Many children never take a pacifier, though, and if you never start with one you will not have to worry about the down-sides. It is not mandatory that a child use one.

Expanding further on this important topic of pacifiers, is important you are not buying into the lie that your baby will use you as a pacifier. Let me make this clear, the pacifier was invented to replace the breast, not the other way around. The pacifier interrupts the biological design, but that does not make it evil. Every time you let your baby suckle at the breast you are providing multiple benefits to both yourself and your baby. They are driven to suckle as much as possible and that is not on accident. It is part of the design of the symbiotic parent-infant relationship. It helps your baby feel connected, cared for, and trusting. It helps the baby's face and palate develop optimally. It helps the postpartum body recover and boosts emotional health. That being said, this is where your discretion and best judgement will come in. It is likely a reasonable choice and low risk option to use the pacifier sparingly. It can also be a helpful tool while working on extending stretches of sleep to a longer duration, or after bottles for soothing to avoid over-feeding.

Sleep Sacks and Swaddles

Babies often love the snug feeling of sleep sacks and swaddles for several reasons. The snuggly feeling is familiar, like when they were cuddled up in the womb. They also keep the baby from startling themselves awake when their limbs spasm in their sleep. Studies have shown that babies get more restful, deeper, and longer sleep sessions in swaddles and sleep sacks. They can be tricky to wean off of, but helpful for the first few months.

After babies can roll over, it is unsafe to continue to swaddle or restrict their use of their arms and legs to roll their body over again as needed. You will need to plan to stop using them. There are versions of sleep sacks that allow for free arm movement, and step by step approaches to stop using the full body versions. Sleep sacks are preferable to swaddling in my opinion due to longevity of use, ability to still show reflexes, as well as avoidance of hip development issues. Sleep sacks and swaddling are not a safe tool to combine with bed-sharing due to risk of over-heating and inability to react protectively if their airway is blocked. They can be a helpful tool to use in conjunction with other tools and methods when trying to get more rest.

Mechanical Bassinets

As technology advances, inventions keep coming out that help babies sleep more. Mechanical bassinets are supposed to be a safe way to get more sleep. Some babies do not respond to them, and they can be an expensive tool. They are a high risk tool when used for a breastfed baby because part of the facts around its use is that utilizing them will often cause parents to miss cues for feeding, and this will potentially sabotage lactation due to missed feeds, especially for younger infants. They might be reasonable to use in shorter increments, and perhaps with an older baby. It reduces risk of lactation sabotage if you are sure to get your baby out to feed often enough (every 2-3 hours and one longer 4-6 hour stretch for an infant past 12 weeks old). If you use them on a very young baby, however, you will be missing critical feeding cues during growth spurts and cluster feeding sessions that are intended to boost and maintain milk supply. They also have weight limits that give them a limited time frame for being useful. When it would be appropriate for an infant to sleep in longer stretches, they have often outgrown these devices' suggested limits. You might use them in conjunction with sleep training methods, or while attempting to adjust sleep cycles. Use your best judgement on these and know the risks.

EVALUATE AND RE-EVALUATE

Once you introduce changes to the nursing and sleeping relationship you should routinely evaluate if it is working for you and for your baby. This section will be full of examples of questions you could ask yourself in evaluation phases. Start with: Is this plan bringing you more stress? Is it causing a lot of tension in the house? Is the baby's growth still on track? Is everyone resting better (as was the goal)?

Weighing an infant who is under 6 months old to evaluate how their growth is tracking once you have introduced a change should take place every 1-2 weeks. An infant older than 6 months can be weighed every 2-4 weeks, but more often if there is a discernable dip in the growth rate (greater than 10 percentile points different), allowing for some variation of growth patterns over time.

With each new phase will come a re-evaluation. Once you get in a groove and figure things out, your baby starts teething, has a mental leap, or goes into a sleep regression. Then you start offering solids. Then they go in and out of even liking eating solids, and they go on and off with how much they like to nurse. What is normal is that there is no normal that lasts the duration of the nursing relationship. It is a dynamic and ever-changing relationship. This is true with infant and young toddler sleep patterns, as well. Many parents are surprised to learn that "sleep-training" is not just done once, but it is done repeatedly with each interruption to sleep routines.

Part of the evaluation should also include other potential reasons for frequent waking outside of what is biologically normal or expected. Does your baby feel dry enough in their particular diaper? Do they have airway anomalies disrupting breathing and causing frequent waking? Do they have untreated reflux that is causing pain and frequent waking? Is the room cool enough, dark enough, and with the right kind of background noise? Does your child have growing pains? Did we pick poor timing to start this? Does your baby like loud white noise or total silence? Are you drinking too much caffeine or having it too late in the day? Does your baby seem to rest better alone, or while sharing a room? What other ways have you tried to facilitate sleep? Are you following your intuition about what is or isn't working, or are you trying to force something that isn't working?

Evaluation and re-evaluation should also include your overall lactation goals. Are you okay with sacrificing a 100% breastmilk diet for more sleep? Is that trade off worth it if it means you will nurse 12 months rather than 6? Do you only prioritize exclusive breastmilk ingestion the first 6 months? Do you want to work in 1 or 2 feedings that your partner handles, to facilitate more rest for you? Can they be pumped milk, donor milk, or formula? These are realistic and logistical questions that you should ask yourself when you evaluate the sleeping and nursing dynamics.

When you evaluate your plan from the beginning, does it include bottles? How will your routine work if you are also working outside of the home? Do you have adequate assistance from other adults? Could you ask more of others? Are there other methods you want to explore? Could you consult a specialist?

Knowing if your baby will take a bottle or not is a common fear for parents who will be working outside of their home within the infant's first year of life. This is a common fear even if you do not have to go back to work, as you will likely want to know in the event of needing to leave the baby that they can be fed. Reasons might be emergent or practical, such as needing to go to an appointment where the baby cannot go with you. I think the best way to handle this is to be proactive, introduce bottles early and often. I know, shocking from an IBCLC but it is true.

I wish I could tell the parents who come to me at 3 to 6 months to go back in time and stay on top of those bottle skills. Introducing 1 or 2 pump sessions and 1 or 2 bottles at least weekly in the early weeks postpartum allows parents to get familiar with the pump, start building a freezer stash, ensure the baby will take a bottle, and allows the lactating parent to get rest and breaks from time to time. I believe avoiding pumps and bottles for the first 6 weeks can be counter-productive to many modern parent's desires and realistic long term logistics of their nursing relationship. Whether or not a lactation consultant wants you to avoid bottles and pumping is, to me, irrelevant. What matters is what the parents want, and what their long-term goals are. I rarely see these steps taken in moderation and under guidance to sabotage the establishment of lactation. In fact, I find the rest that is facilitated for the feeding parent makes them more likely to continue to nurse than if they were exhausted and worn down without ever being given a chance to get a break or have a stretch of sleep longer than 2-3 hours for months on end.

The biological norm is to breastfeed, and an older baby is perfectly happy to do so when it is all they know. There is absolutely nothing wrong with keeping with this biological norm. However, when you need to return to work when they are 3-6 months old, they will not understand the desire to introduce the bottle, nor see the need. Most consultants will have some helpful tricks for you to get the baby to take a bottle, but do yourself a favor and let them have one early and often if you know they will likely ever need one in the first 6 months of life. Bottles offered can be snacks, just 1 to 2 ounces, and do not necessarily need to be a full feed. The flexibility of feeding method is a great stress reducer for most parents. If we miss our opportunity or baby loses the bottle-feeding skill, then after 6 months we can move on to sippy cups, straw cups, and lots of solids when a parent has to be away. The bottle should be offered at least weekly, as sometimes a baby that takes bottles fine the first 2 months can lose the skill and then refuse it when offered again months later.

There can be some other logistical challenges to sleep training and lactation in general when the lactating parent and infant are separated for many of the waking hours during the week. Nursing less throughout the night might mean over-all reducing time or opportunities for nursing. This might make the parent sad. So sad, they find they would rather lose sleep than lose out on nursing sessions. Many infants "reverse cycle" and will nurse more frequently when the parent is home to make up for the lost time apart. They may be reluctant to give up that time at the breast, and refuse bottles during the day. If a parent is not particularly responsive to pumping, supply may also suffer. Additionally, the infant may not cooperate. These are just things to consider, and it is still okay to choose to move forward despite these inherent risks to the lactation relationship.

Be aware of the possibility that your infant might need an underlying issue addressed before getting more rest can be facilitated. If your infant has had poor sleep with frequent wakinge very 1-2 hours for longer than a few weeks it might be an issue that needs addressed medically, and not a sleep issue. Babies should be able to be soothed back to sleep, even with frequent waking. Look to how your baby behaves during the day, too. If they are hard to soothe day and night, there might be a different issue to address. If you just aren't sure, utilize your resources and consult your medical team. This includes the baby's provider and your IBCLC, and maybe others.

We can make all the plans in the world, between you and me, but there is still a third party here that has to go along with these new plans (the baby). In addition to that, our bodies may respond differently than we expect them to. Some lactating people can tolerate nursing or pumping less frequently, and still make a full supply. These are things you will likely not know the answer to until you make the commitment and go through the trial and error process. Consider working with a sleep consultant if you are really struggling.

Other helpful lactation information:

For a more in-depth explanation of concepts introduced in this text, lactation relationship norms, potential problems, how mental health relates to our nursing relationships, and much more, see my lactation book "Can I talk you out of breastfeeding? A quick guide to everything that can be challenging about breastfeeding" available on audible, kindle, and paperback through Kindle Direct Publishing.

This tongue-in-cheek book has the educational material modern parents are craving. Tired of hearing parents felt unprepared for the realities of lactation (or infant feeding in general) I seek to change the conversations we have around lactation. As a low supply mother, Family Nurse Practitioner and Board Certified Lactation Consultant with an additional degree in psychology, I have a lot to add to the dialogue. Covering topics no other lactation book dares, this is more than a how-to manual and gives real and practical information. Mental health is at the forefront of this inclusive and dynamic book that covers all the challenges and all the options and gives the information that parents actually want. This book seeks to empower parents to make the best personalized decisions for their families from an informed space. Resources for when you hit snags included! It makes a great gift for expectant parents, especially.

Follow me @thelactationpractitioner on Facebook and Instagram for relevant content and news, and new book announcements. You will also find a link there to book with me for a virtual consult if you need some guidance.

If you enjoyed this book and learned from it, please leave me a review through the platform that you purchased the book from and recommend it to your friends.

RESOURCES

You should have a healthcare team set up to help you face potential challenges. Start with meeting with an IBCLC. Choose a breastfeeding supportive pediatrician. Ask them questions about what ways they support breastfeeding, and make sure their ideals match yours. Bring in a speech and language pathologist, and myofunctional therapist and body workers like massage therapists, chiropractors and cranial sacral therapists as needed for feeding difficulties. Have an idea of who you would talk to or go see if you feel you needed emotional or mental health support. Ask around your local community for recommendations of these specialists. Build your healthcare village.

Remember that everyone you know is a resource. Your support circle needs to grow, and you should be the one to grow it. Do not wait for people to volunteer, tell them how they can help. When people do offer to help, tell them something specific you want. If someone is willing to do something for you, let them.

Additionally, my lactation book is a great resource for navigating this time because I cover many topics that others leave out such as your relationships with others, returning to work, low supply, pumping, supplementing, introducing solids, and much, much more.

Do not forget the amazing resource of technology that we have as modern parents. You can get many free apps on your phone to track feedings, diapers, sleep, measurements, and milestones. You can utilize social media and search engines for many things, as long as you also consult your professional team. Social media can also be very beneficial to combatting isolation and loneliness, as it can connect you with other parents. You can send pictures and video-chat with family if you do not want to have them over, or if they live too far to visit. You can also attend online classes, do online prenatal consults, have an online sleep consultation, attend online support groups, and watch how-to videos of many of the hands-on skills you will need like pumping, swaddling, and burping.

You are also a powerful resource unto yourself. You can do a lot to prepare. Go to a prenatal consult. Take the parenting and breastfeeding classes, read the books, do the meal-prep, freeze some padsicles, and do the mental and emotional work. Manage your own expectations. Take responsibility for yourself by asking for help and setting boundaries. Give yourself grace, compassion, and patience. Trust your instincts. Seek help early and often.

Find an IBCLC

You need support from a local or virtual IBCLC. When you see a lactation consultant, like myself, I suggest a prenatal lactation assessment to review your risk factors and take steps specific to your risks to maximize your supply before pregnancy, during, and immediately postpartum. They can help in the early weeks and up until weaning, even if that is well into childhood. I, personally, am available for virtual consults and local in-person consults.

Even without some of the problems mentioned in my lactation book, lactation is generally challenging. Becoming a new parent is challenging. Lean into your community and reach out for help. Do not wait until there is a problem; see an IBCLC before pregnancy, during, and after. Let them monitor your progress in those fragile early weeks. Let them help you troubleshoot, perfect, and optimize your lactation experience.

I am available virtually, find me on Instagram @thelactationpractitioner and I will have the best way to book with me in my bio. Local appointments may be available and might be covered by insurance if you are on the Olympic Peninsula in Washington State.

Utilize your lactation benefits through insurance (USA specific)

The Affordable Healthcare Act, signed into law in 2010, ensures that more females in the United States have access to coverage for lactation support and pumping equipment. As of the writing of this book in 2020, this is still in effect. Health insurance plans, outside of grandfathered plans and certain state Medicaid plans, must provide lactation support and equipment for the duration of lactation, and some help is available during pregnancy. This means you are able to get a prenatal lactation consult, and possibly get your pump before baby comes. The pump provided might be a rental, manual, or electric. Some require birth of the baby before they will issue the pump. It should be up to you and your provider which option is best for you, and they can write a prescription to be filled by a medical supply company. Some plans cover other equipment like bags or valve replacements, or they are at least FSA/HSA (Flexible Spending or Healthcare Spending accounts) eligible. Much of the nursing and pumping paraphernalia is covered under FSA/HSA spending, so always check before you purchase or check if you are eligible for reimbursement. The equipment offered may require partial cost-sharing if you choose to upgrade, but a no-cost option should also be available. The lactation support might need to be with an in-network provider, require prior-authorization, or referral. Lactation services are considered preventative medicine, as lactation is a biological expectation, and you should not have any co-pays, payments toward deductible, or co-insurance fees. If you see an OB/GYN, CNM, pediatrician, or FNP (like me) who is also an IBCLC you might be covered under preventative medicine as well, and this may not count towards using the lactation consult benefit. This is important to know if your plan places a limit on number of visits per year. This is information you want to clarify while you are still pregnant so you can plan ahead and have help lined up for when you inevitably need it. If you are outside of the USA call your health plan to ask what lactation support can be expected.

If you are in the USA, here is a helpful toolkit to help you understand your rights under this law, and suggestions to hold your plan accountable if they are not meeting the standards set forth by the law. https://www.nwlc.org/sites/default/files/pdfs/final_nwlcbreastfeedingtoolkit2014_edit.pdf

Find an oral tether/tongue tie provider

If you suspect your child has oral tethers it is best to find a "preferred provider" with a reputation for doing thorough work. Follow up with finding stretches and exercises for oral tethers; you can start these even before a revision. This is where you will want to involve your healthcare village. https://www.tt-lt-support-network.com/

There are also many Facebook support groups, usually separated by state, where you can get feedback from other parents who have seen providers in your area. They also typically share how their recovery process was, and other associated therapists, consultants, and bodyworkers in the area that aided in their post-procedure recovery and functional optimization.

Infant Risk
This is the resource I mentioned previously for what medication is safe during pregnancy and breastfeeding. They have a website, app, book, and hotline. https://www.infantrisk.com/

Jack Newman, M.D. Breastfeeding Medicine Specialist Jack Newman's website is an excellent resource for breastfeeding information. Visit https://www.breastfeedinginc.ca/

Mother-Baby Behavioral Sleep Lab, University of Notre Dame, Dr. James McKenna "Safe Infant Sleep" by James J McKenna, Ph.D. https://cosleeping.nd.edu/

PPD/PPA Resources
Postpartum Support International: https://www.postpartum.net/ Warm Line (non-emergent phone support): 1 800 944 4773

Postpartum Support International offers phone support, online chat support, online support meetings and local resources. Online support meetings are held weekly for both moms and dads. Information is available at this site in both English and Spanish.

Text HOME to 741741 if you need immediate assistance you can find help 24 hours a day, 7 days a week and have a cell phone and are in the United States. Their website explains their services. https://www.crisistextline.org/text-us/

Call the National Suicide Prevention Hotline: 1800 273 8255, also available 24/7

Domestic Abuse Resources

National Domestic Violence Hotline, which has a website with education and resources, as well as a chat feature, in addition to their hotline phone number. https://www.thehotline.org/ When you go to the website you will be prompted with this warning: "Internet usage can be monitored and is impossible to erase completely. If you are concerned your internet usage might be monitored, call us at 1 800 799 SAFE (7233). Learn more about digital security and remember to clear your browser history after visiting this website. Click the "X" or "Escape" button at any time to leave TheHotline.org immediately."

Kellymom website, breastfeeding and parenting guide https://kellymom.com/

National Women's Law Center "Breastfeeding Students" pamphlet FAQs https://nwlc.org/wp-content/uploads/2016/08/FAQBreastfeeding_nwlc_PPToolkitAug2016.pdf

Substance Abuse and Mental Health Services Administration 1-800-662-4357
https://www.samhsa.gov/find-help/national-helpline

Bedsharing and Breastfeeding: The Academy of Breastfeeding Medicine Protocol #6, Revision 2019
https://www.bfmed.org/assets/Protocol%20Number%206%202019%20Revision.pdf

Red Nose. National Scientific Advisory Group (NSAG). (2015 May). Information Sheet: Sleeping with a baby. Melbourne, National SIDs Council of Australia. Last updated December 2019.
https://rednose.org.au/downloads/
InfoStatement_SharingSleepSurfacewithBaby_Dec2019.pdf

Basis, Infant Sleep Info Source, UK.
https://www.basisonline.org.uk/

AFTERWORD

If you enjoyed this book and feel like you learned from it I would appreciate feedback in the form of a review on the platform you purchased from, and do please share it with others who you think would benefit from the knowledge shared here.

www.ingramcontent.com/pod-product-compliance
Lightning Source LLC
Chambersburg PA
CBHW061514250726
48657CB00005B/1857